MOSBY'S
Assessment
Memory
NoteCards

Visual, Mnemonic, and
Memory Aids for Nurses

JoAnn Zerwekh, EdD, RN, FNP, APRN, BC

Executive Director
Nursing Education Consultants
Ingram, Texas

Nursing Faculty – Online Campus
University of Phoenix
Phoenix, Arizona

Tom Gaglione, RN, MSN
Nursing Faculty
Nursing Education Consultants
Ingram, Texas

C.J. Miller, BSN, RN
Illustrator
Nursing Education Consultants
Washington, Iowa

Reviewed by

Ashlov Zerwekh, DN, DA

Monograph content contributed by

MSN, RN, PhD

ector of Nursing
n College
cius, Minnesota

MOSBY
ELSEVIER

MOSBY
ELSEVIER

11830 Westline Industrial Drive
St. Louis, Missouri 63146

MOSBY'S ASSESSMENT
MEMORY NOTECARDS: VISUAL,
MNEMONIC, AND MEMORY AIDS
FOR NURSES

ISBN-13: 978-0-323-04403-5
ISBN-10:-0-323-04403-4

NOTICE

Nursing is an ever-changing field. Standard safety precautions must be followed, but
as new research and clinical experience broaden our knowledge, changes in treatment
and drug therapy may become necessary or appropriate. Readers are advised to check
the most current product information provided by the manufacturer of each drug to be
administered to verify the recommended dose, the method and duration of administration,
and contraindications. It is the responsibility of the licensed prescriber, relying on experience and knowledge of the patient, to determine dosages and the best treatment for each
individual patient. Neither the publisher nor the author assumes any liability for any injury
and/or damage to persons or property arising from this publication.

ISBN-13: 978-0-323-04403-5
ISBN-10: 0-323-04403-4

Executive Publisher: Robin Carter
Developmental Editor: Deanna Davis
Publishing Services Manager: Jeff Patterson
Senior Book Designer: Julia Dummitt
Cover Art: CJ Miller

Printed in China

Last digit is the print number: 9 8 7 6 5 4 3 2

Working together to grow
libraries in developing countries

www.elsevier.com | www.bookaid.org | www.sabre.org

ELSEVIER   BOOK AID
            International   Sabre Foundation

Contents

GENERAL TYPES OF ASSESSMENT

OBTAINING HEALTH INFORMATION

PHYSICAL ASSESSMENT

Contents

ASSESSMENT CONSIDERATIONS ACROSS THE LIFESPAN

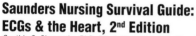

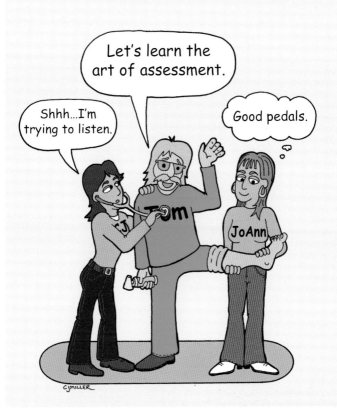

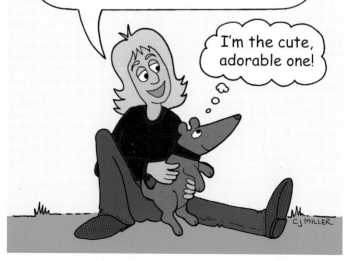

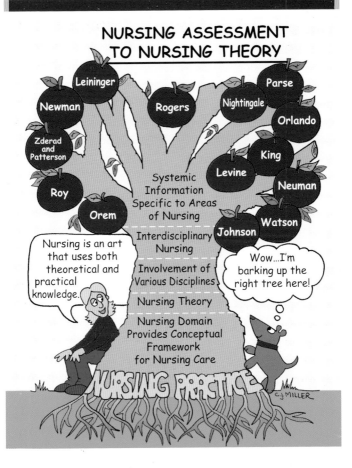

Assessment at a Glance
Nursing Assessment to Nursing Theory

As a professional nurse, the basis for an assessment must be chosen.
- How does the nurse know which body systems to include in the health history or physical examination? When should the health history and physical examination begin?
- Answers to these questions are dependent on many factors. The nurse must have a theoretical foundation for the care he or she is providing.
- Choosing a theory that is congruent with the mission of the health care organization will assist in meeting the client's needs.

ADEQUATE EVALUATION

- A theory-based assessment ensures that the nurse will adequately evaluate the client, his or her current situation, and the overall circumstances.
- If a sound framework is not in place, then the nurse risks missing vital information on which the entire plan of care is based.
- The choice of theory depends on who the client is, the health care environment, and, to a certain degree, the nurse or organization that is providing the care.

THEORISTS

Orlando	Theory of Deliberative Nursing Process
Levine	Conservation Model
Rogers	Science of Unitary Human Beings
Orem	Self-Care Nursing Theory
King	Theory of Goal Attainment
Neuman	Neuman Systems Model
Roy	Roy's Adaptation Model
Paterson & Zderad	Humanistic Nursing Theory
Leininger	Theory of Culture Care Diversity and Universality
Newman	Theory of Health as Expanding Consciousness
Watson	Theory of Human Caring
Johnson	Behavioral Systems Model
Parse	Theory of Human Becoming
Nightingale	No name to her model

Important nursing implications	Abnormal findings
Common clinical findings	Patient teaching

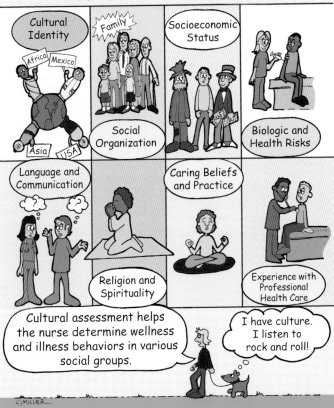

Assessment at a Glance
Cultural Assessment

Culture may dictate:
- Client's predisposition to disease (Native Americans, diabetes)
- Client's perception of health care ("Only wimps go to the doctor...")
- Language spoken
  Culture alone cannot completely describe any one individual, family, or group.

ASSESSMENT CONSIDERATIONS

- Ask the client whether any special health care practices, herbal treatments, or dietary considerations should be noted.
- These considerations may include situations such as:
  - Men answering all the questions for the women
  - Preference for women practitioners for female clients
  - Family shouting through most conversations
  - Belief that blood products are not acceptable treatments
  - Belief that asking questions is a sign of weakness or disrespect

  Pursuing cultural competence through continued study (nursing journals, web sites) will improve the nurse's ability to identify cultural characteristics.

CLIENT PERCEPTIONS

- The nurse should closely assess for client perceptions in all situations.
- Collecting these data will not only improve care planning, but it will also open up the lines of communication between the client and nurse. Taking an interest and demonstrating to the client that his or her opinions are valuable will foster a sense of mutual trust.

BE SELF-AWARE

- The nurse must understand his or her own cultural characteristics and perceptions. The social organization of the nurse's family, as well as the nurse's religious practices and socioeconomic status, will affect the way the nurse responds to clients.

Important nursing implications	Abnormal findings
Common clinical findings	Patient teaching

COMMUNITY ASSESSMENT

Comes in Three Areas

Structure	Population	Social System

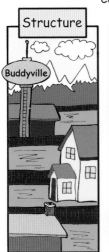
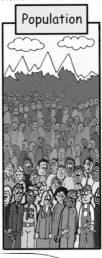
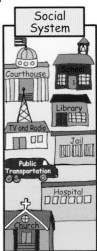

Understanding the makeup of a client's community can help create a more comprehensive picture of the client's health.

A great town with a great name... BUDDYVILLE!

Assessment at a Glance
Community Assessment

Communities can create an environment that affects the health of all members in some way.

STRUCTURE

Geography, climate, and local architectural practices all affect the health of individuals.
- Will the wind carry the pollutants away, or does the air in town stand still?
- How close are potential hazards such as landfills and military proving grounds?
- Is there industry nearby that may contaminate or alter certain food supplies?

POPULATION

Knowing the general composition of the population is important.
- Certain diseases such as hepatitis A and pertussis can be found in greater concentrations in certain populations.
- The population may be very mobile to the point that disease in a population on one continent could affect populations on other continents (severe acute respiratory syndrome [SARS]).
- Does the population have a high concentration of one particular ethnicity that is predisposed to a certain health concern?
- Does a subgroup of a population have certain practices that could become a health issue (growing its own mushrooms)?

SOCIAL SYSTEM

Clients are also affected by the social system in which they live.
- Local governments may provide free health care to certain groups.
- Schools can create a climate that supports health (food choices in the vending machines, health screening programs) or cause difficulties for clients (student with asthma may not carry his or her inhaler to class).
- Community may promote health through screening events at libraries or churches.

Important nursing implications	Abnormal findings
Common clinical findings	Patient teaching

ASSESSMENT OF THE COMMUNITY— WINDSHIELD SURVEY

Information Highway—Windshield Survey

Use your eyes...What and who do you see?

Use your ears...What do you hear?

Use your nose...What do you smell?

Use combined senses to feel around you mentally and physically.

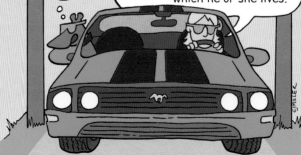

Road trip, road trip! Burgers and fries!

The best way to understand your client's condition is to understand the environment in which he or she lives. Driving to and from your client's residence allows you to assess the area in which he or she lives.

Assessment at a Glance
Assessment of the Community—Windshield Survey

A great deal of data can be collected as the nurse moves through the community. While driving to a client's house, the nurse will see, hear, and smell many things that can offer important clues. The nurse will synthesize this information to assist in developing the plan of care. The nurse will need to triangulate information gathered from the windshield survey to data collection from the health history and physical assessment.

KEY CONCEPTS

- Neighborhood
  - Housing—state of repair, number of multifamily units (apartments, condominiums, duplexes), mobile home parks, vacant lots, vacant buildings
  - Parks and nature—green spaces, state parks, forests, trees, public parks, private parks, vandalism
  - Hangouts and public places (commons)—benches in front of the barbershop, cars parked in vacant lots with many people congregating, teenagers at the drive-in theater
- Services
  - Schools—state of repair, old or new, fenced off, police and security guards
  - Commerce—stores, banks, electric companies, gas stations; state of repair, bars on the windows, litter, vandalism
  - Public works and services—fire hydrants intact, library, fire, police
  - Charity—Salvation Army, homeless shelters, churches
- Population
  - Race and ethnicity—homogenous, heterogeneous, minorities
  - Homelessness—people sleeping in alleys, on steps, or park benches
  - Health and well being—children appear well-nourished and clean, number of free clinics, number of "soup kitchens"
- Transportation
  - Walking, public transportation (bus, subway; state of repair), automobiles (new, old; state of repair)

Important nursing implications	Abnormal findings
Common clinical findings	Patient teaching

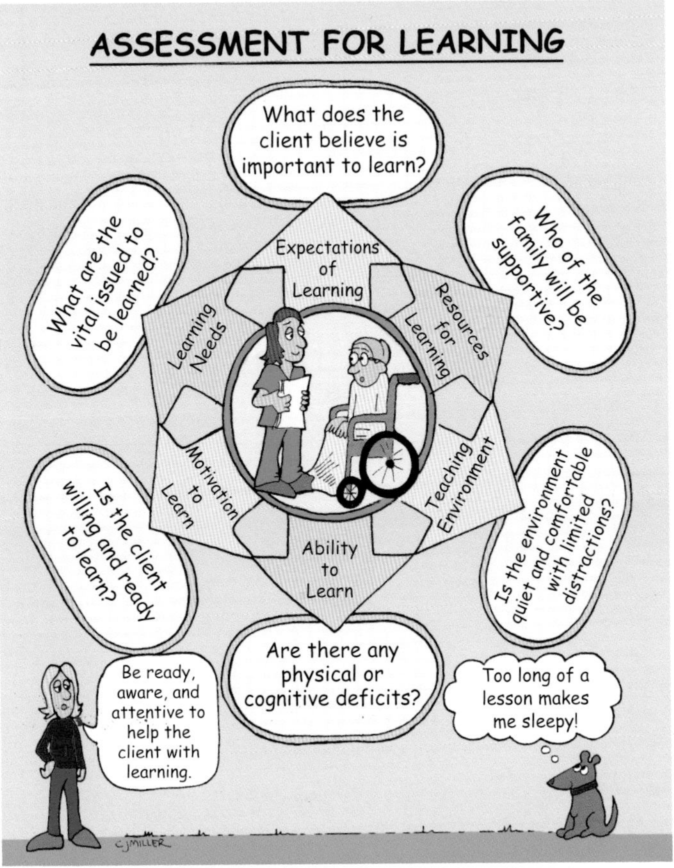
ASSESSMENT FOR LEARNING
What does the client believe is important to learn?
Who of the family will be supportive?
Is the environment quiet and comfortable with limited distractions?
Are there any physical or cognitive deficits?
Is the client willing and ready to learn?
What are the vital issued to be learned?
Expectations of Learning
Resources for Learning
Teaching Environment
Ability to Learn
Motivation to Learn
Learning Needs
Be ready, aware, and attentive to help the client with learning.
Too long of a lesson makes me sleepy!
C.J.MILLER

Assessment at a Glance
Assessment for Learning

As the nurse collects data about the physical and psychologic status of the client, assessment of his or her learning needs is important.
- Understanding the need for learning is important because it could affect the client's ability to provide adequate data.
- Identifying and addressing learning needs will also affect the client's ability to understand and implement the plan of care.

OPPORTUNITY

Nurses should look for opportunities to include health care–related information to the client and family throughout the physical exams and other assessments events.

READINESS

Before learning can begin, the nurse needs to assess the client for readiness.
- Ability to learn (vision, hearing, intellectual status, language barriers)
- Motivation ("If I quit smoking, I will gain weight…")
- Comfort (pain, distress, nicotine withdrawal)

Learning materials may need to be altered to meet certain needs (vision, hearing, translator).

ENVIRONMENT

- Issues such as television, family members, and other distractions can hinder the client's ability to learn or the nurse's ability to teach.
- Care should be taken to assess the environment before the learning interaction begins with adjustments made accordingly.

CLIENT NEEDS

- The nurse may identify multiple learning needs (smoking, obesity, domestic violence) that need to be prioritized.
- Trying to meet all the client's learning needs in one encounter will often cause the client to feel overwhelmed and will decrease the effectiveness of the teaching.

Important nursing implications	Abnormal findings
Common clinical findings	Patient teaching

ASSESSMENT OF STRESS AND COPING

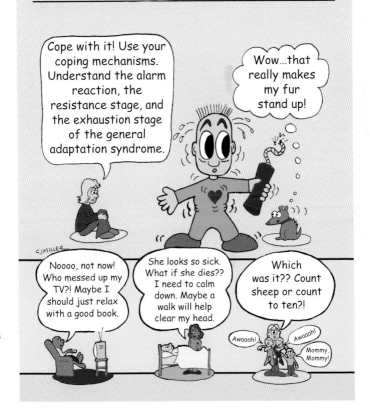

Assessment at a Glance
Assessment of Stress and Coping

Understanding the client's response to stress and the subsequent coping mechanisms are important for effective health assessment.

- Stress affects multiple body systems and psychologic processes.
- The affects can be seen throughout the data collection phase of the assessment.

GENERAL ADAPTATION SYNDROME (GAS)

- Alarm reaction (varied degrees of fight or flight)
- Resistance (return to normal functioning and repair)
- Exhaustion (stress persists, resistance is eventually no longer maintained).
  The physiologic responses of GAS can hide, mimic, or intensify health assessment findings related to other issues, which may make data collection difficult because certain signs or symptoms may not be apparent.

IMMUNE SYSTEM

- Suppression of the immune system is another issue to consider.

COPING

Stress is going to affect everyone at some time.
- For many individuals, coping is effective and can allow for effective resistance and repair (walks on the beach).
- For others, coping is destructive and leads to even more stress (turning to abusive relationships, using alcohol or drugs).
- The nurse needs to collect data about the client's coping practices.
- Coping mechanisms will provide the nurse with valuable information about learning needs. Finally, coping mechanisms may also provide the client with effective solutions to current and future health care needs.

Important nursing implications	Abnormal findings
Common clinical findings	Patient teaching

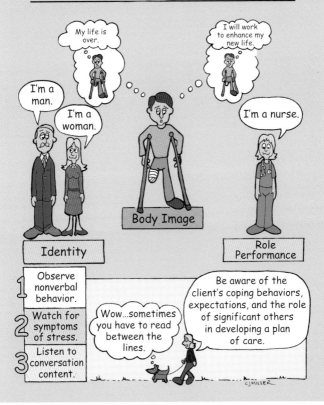

Assessment at a Glance
Assessment of Self-Concept

Self-concept is the perception that an individual holds of him or herself and includes the client's body image, identity, and role performance. Each individual, no matter how similar his or her characteristics are, will have a unique self-concept.

BODY IMAGE

- Varies greatly and is multifactorial in nature.
- Amputation, mastectomy, and other surgeries or injuries (burns) may affect a client's body image.

The nurse must identify the individual's self-concept and determine how it affects the client's overall health. Questions to consider include:

- What does this mean to you and your family and friends?
- What is your greatest strength? Greatest weakness?
- What would you like to change about yourself?

Answers to these questions, nonverbal cues during the interview, and other information will provide important data for the nurse to identify the client's self-concept.

IDENTITY AND ROLE PERFORMANCE

Another key component of self-concept is, "Who do you say you are?"

- Self-identity can be a part of gender orientation, religious affiliation, or social group.
- During the assessment of the client's perceptions about these areas, certain clues may arise as to how the person's self-concept may affect his or her health.

Role performance can also have a significant influence.

- May include profession, vocation, civic service, or group identity.

| Important nursing implications | Abnormal findings |
| Common clinical findings | Patient teaching |

SPIRITUAL ASSESSMENT

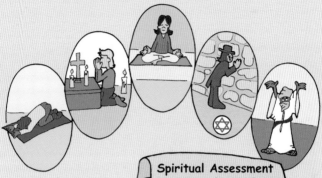

Spiritual Assessment
- Assess client's faith and beliefs.
- Determine whether the client practices religious rituals.
- Assess the extent of the client's fellowship within the community.

The nurse must not color a client's spiritual assessment by his or her own spiritual beliefs. Be self-aware during this type of assessment.

Assessment at a Glance
Spiritual Assessment

Nurses need to identify spiritual characteristics of the client.

BE SELF-AWARE

The nurse must understand his or her own spiritual beliefs and perceptions and acknowledge core beliefs to address responses that may adversely affect his or her therapeutic interaction with a client.

VARIATION IN INDIVIDUALS

As with other parts of sociocultural assessment, individuals within a group may vary greatly.
The nurse needs to identify what religion and spirituality means to each client.

ASSESSMENT PROCESS

Many assessment forms address spirituality by simply asking whether the client would like a member of the clergy to visit. Although this question is important, it is far from adequate. Data collection should include:
- Faith, denomination, and tradition
- Client's level of agreement with his or her faith
- Client's level of service and level of practice (rituals) in his or her faith
- Client's social network related to his or her faith

FEAR AND SPIRITUALITY

- Many clients do not think of spirituality until they are involved in a health-altering experience, which places important responsibility on the nurse to consider ways in which the client's perceptions of spiritual concepts may affect his or her health.
- Nurses need to assess the client related to his or her fear and ask questions about spiritual perceptions. If more assistance is needed, then clergy consultation may be indicated.

Important nursing implications	Abnormal findings
Common clinical findings	Patient teaching

GRIEF AND LOSS ASSESSMENT

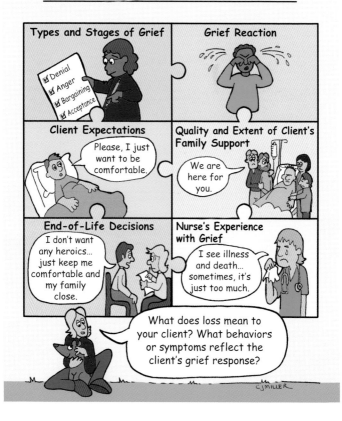

=== Assessment at a Glance ===
Grief and Loss Assessment

When loss occurs, whether real or perceived, a bond is severed between the loss (relationship, health, status, something symbolic) and the individual. Nurses need to identify the meaning associated with loss and assist the client in coping.

GRIEF RESPONSE

Loss initiates the grief response and varies among individuals, but most clients will go through the various stages that include:
- Denial—is sometimes referred to as numbing or ignoring the situation
- Anger—is usually displaced
- Bargaining—not fully accepting; thinking that there must be a way out
- Depression—feelings of hopelessness, weariness, and loneliness
- Acceptance—understanding what has happened and is able to function normally

The nurse has a responsibility to identify the stage through which the client may be passing and assess for the potential effects of that stage on outcomes.

DEATH AND DYING

- Nurses should be comfortable with addressing end-of-life decisions.
- Client and family expectations are assessed in end-of-life situations.
- Creating a therapeutic relationship with the client will improve the nurse's ability to speak openly with the client.
- Nurses need to understand the perceptions, structure, and issues of the family members to ensure that their needs are being met.

BE SELF-AWARE

- Nurses need to remember that they are not "super human," which means that the nurse should acknowledge his or her personal strengths and weaknesses concerning death and dying.
- Nurses should discuss death and dying with others to ensure that they are not repressing emotions that should be addressed.
- The nurse's feelings and internal struggles can affect the client's care.

| Important nursing implications | Abnormal findings |
| Common clinical findings | Patient teaching |

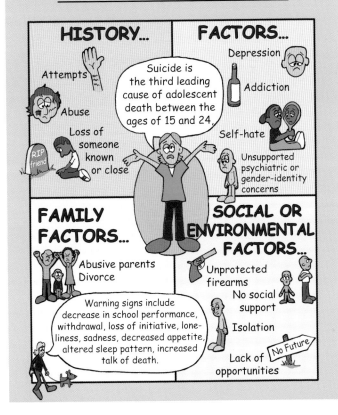

Assessment at a Glance
Suicide Risk Assessment

Nurses have a serious responsibility to be alert to the warning signs of suicide by identifying certain flags that warrant further investigation. If a flag is identified, then the client should be asked directly whether he or she has any thoughts of harming him or herself.

HISTORY

- A previous suicide attempt is an important issue that warrants investigation.
- Children who have been abused may adopt a self-concept of worthlessness that leads to a decision to commit suicide.
- Significant losses of family or friends can also precipitate suicide.

FACTORS

- Depression is often involved and can be related to chronic illness.
- Does the client have an altered self image? Is there an addiction?
- Other issues include a lack of support from significant others.

FAMILY FACTORS

- When stress at home becomes too great, clients may view suicide as a means of release or escape.
- Clients at high risk may come from families who have struggled with domestic violence and divorce, which should be considered a flag for the nurse.

SOCIAL AND ENVIRONMENTAL FACTORS

- Are there unsecured firearms available to the client?
- Is the client isolated or unsupported by family or friends or both?

WARNING SIGNS

- Decreased performance, withdrawal, loneliness
- Loss of initiative, sadness, decreased appetite
- Altered sleep pattern, increased talk of death

Important nursing implications	Abnormal findings
Common clinical findings	Patient teaching

COMMUNICATION ASSESSMENT

Assessment at a Glance
Communication Assessment

KEY CONCEPTS

- Physical and Emotional Factors
  - Neurologic—Uses expressive or receptive communication (stroke, mental retardation).
  - Sensory—is deaf or blind (unable to see nonverbal signs).
  - Critically ill or short of breath—Spaces out the discussions, questioning, yes-and-no questions.
  - Emotional illness comes in many different forms.
    - Aggressiveness—Client and nurse safety are priorities.
    - Prioritize—Most important information is gathered first.
    - Confusion—Collaborate with family.
- Developmental Factors
  - Infant—Crying indicates a need (fear, food, pain, comfort).
    - Build rapport with parent; exhibit firm, calm, and slow handling of infant.
  - Child—Refer to a child by name.
    - Build rapport with the parent, then include the child.
    - With younger children, spend more time in the beginning "ignoring" them to allow the children to observe you.
  - Adolescent—Do not talk down to them.
    - Include the parent when appropriate.
  - Older adult—Address him or her directly, even when the family is present.
    - Maintain respectful, slow, low tones of speech to facilitate clear understanding.
    - Avoid rushing.
- Sociocultural Factors
  - Maintain eye level when communicating with no barriers (desk).
  - Gender
    - Avoid humor, innuendos; maintain personal space.
    - Acknowledge gender issues.

Important nursing implications	Abnormal findings
Common clinical findings	Patient teaching

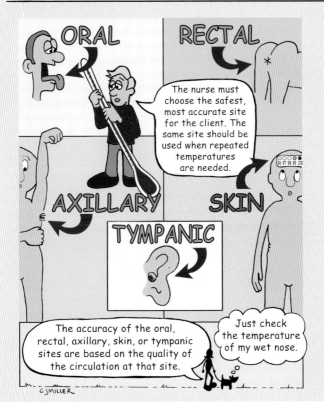

Assessment at a Glance
Assessment of Thermoregulation

NORMAL RANGE OF FINDINGS

- Heat production and loss
  - Production and conservation—shivering
  - Loss—sweating, peripheral vasodilation
- Normal range
  - Adult—37° C (98.6° F); older adult—36.2° C (97.2° F)
  - Infant—wide fluctuation because of immature thermoregulation
- Routes
  - Tympanic—May be affected by the environment; may be less accurate in client who is under age 6 years.
  - Oral—Wait 15 minutes after the intake of food or drink, 2 minutes after smoking; place thermometer in the posterior sublingual pocket; instruct patient to keep lips closed.
  - Rectal—Adult: wear gloves, lubricate, insert 1 inch, red probes and thermometers are usually rectal.
  - Axillary—Effective at room temperature.
  - Skin—Thermometer strips are not accurate and should not be used if the room temperature is over 39° C.
- Electronic—Is it charged? Calibrated?
- Women—Increases 0.5° to 1.0° F with ovulation.

ABNORMAL FINDINGS

- Adult—Diurnal—1.0° to 1.5° F higher in the afternoon.
  - Neurologic damage can reset the thermostat.
- Older adult
  - Has a lower febrile response to illness; is a poor gauge of health.
- Children
  - Fevers in response to illness are higher than they are in adults.

Important nursing implications	Abnormal findings
Common clinical findings	Patient teaching

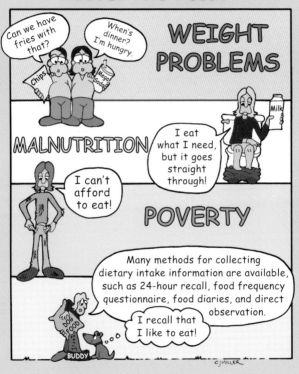

Assessment at a Glance
Assessment of Nutritional Issues and Needs

NORMAL RANGE OF FINDINGS

- Infants and children—Growth charts need to be maintained to ensure proper growth.
  - Not recommended to use skim or low-fat milks ($1/2$% and 1%).
- Adolescent—Need balanced diet, exercise, and rest.
- Adult—Body mass index (BMI) is between 18.5 and 24.9.
  - Older adult
  - Decrease energy requirements are caused by a loss of lean body mass and an increase in fat mass.

ABNORMAL FINDINGS

- Infants and children
  - Anemia can occur as a result of low-iron diets.
- Adolescent
  - Obsession with body image may lead to dangerous habits such as vomiting, excessive exercise, and isolation.
  - Approximately 15% of children and adolescents are overweight.
- Adult
  - Obesity is a serious issue for many adults.
  - Birth of an infant over 10 pounds may be a sign of potential development of diabetes in the mother after the pregnancy.
- Older adult
  - Increase of more than 2 pounds in 1 day may indicate exacerbation of heart failure.
  - Poverty leads many older adults with the tough choice between food and medications. Cheaper food often has lower nutritional value.

Important nursing implications	Abnormal findings
Common clinical findings	Patient teaching

ASSESSMENT OF SLEEP—QUESTIONS

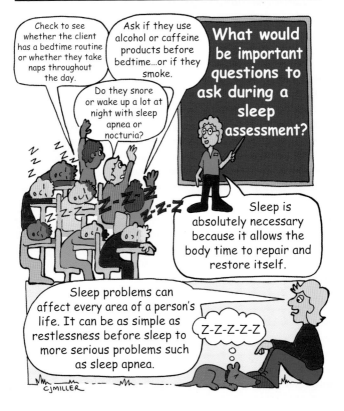

Assessment at a Glance
Assessment of Sleep—Questions

NORMAL RANGE OF FINDINGS

- Neonates—16 hours per day; 2 to 3 hours of sleep, followed by 50 minutes of wake time
- Infants—15 hours per day; 8 to 10 hour stretch at night
- Children—10 to 12 hours per day; naps usually stop at 3 to 4 years of age
- Adolescents—8 hours per day
- Adults and older adults—6 to 8 hours per day; frequent complaints of insomnia (older)

KEY CONCEPTS

- Sleep deprivation—Results from:
  - Physical illness—pain, hypertension, nocturia, dyspnea (sleep apnea), altered positioning (in traction), endocrine disorders, restless leg syndrome
  - Psychologic illness—anxiety, depression, insomnia, alcoholism
- Sleep deprivation—Leads to:
  - Hypertension, heart disease, stroke, sudden death
- Other sleep disorders and concerns
  - Enuresis, sudden infant death syndrome, nightmares and terrors, sleep walking (somnambulism), sleep talking, narcolepsy (sudden sleep attack)

ASSESSMENT QUESTIONS

- Bedtime routine? Sleep schedule (naps)? Snoring?
- Use of alcohol, caffeine, tobacco, controlled substances, other medications throughout the day and night?
- Medications for sleep (diphenhydramine, cough syrup, narcotics, herbals)?
- Number of hours of sleep (start-to-stop and any interruptions)?
- Sleep apnea (choking or shortness of breath, number of pillows used)?
- Sleep positions, furniture ("I sleep in a recliner every night...")?
- Locations, environment (television, other people, lighting)

| Important nursing implications | Abnormal findings |
| Common clinical findings | Patient teaching |

ASSESSMENT OF SLEEP—PHYSICAL ASSESSMENT

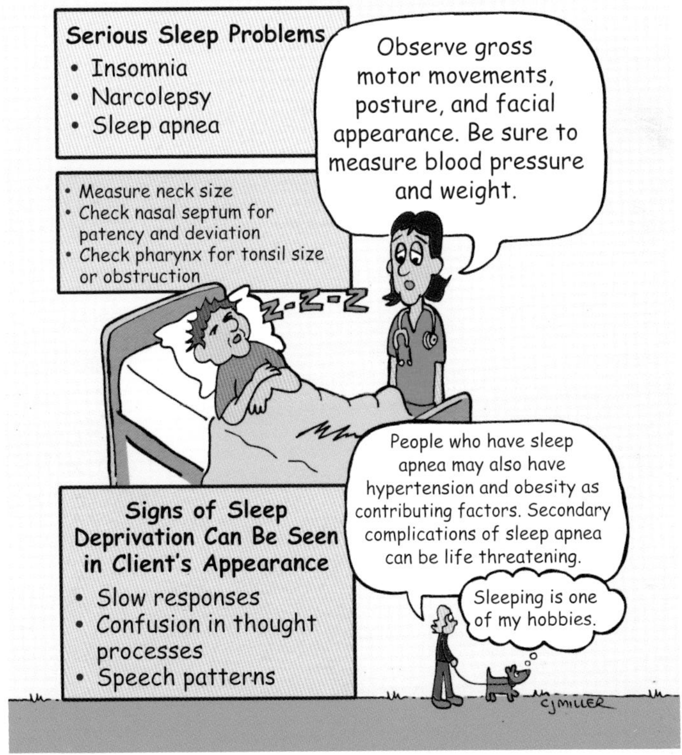

=== Assessment at a Glance ===
Assessment of Sleep—Physical Assessment

The nurse needs to include the signs and symptoms of sleep deprivation in his or her teaching.

KEY CONCEPTS

- Signs and symptoms of sleep deprivation
  - Client appearance—slow responses, confusion, speech patterns
  - Client actions—slow response, range from hyperactive to sleepy, agitated, fine motor impairment
  - Physical assessment—diminished reflexes, ptosis, blurred vision, cardiac arrhythmias
- Diagnostic findings
  - Electroencephalogram (EEG) and electromyogram (EMG).
  - Electrooculogram (EOG)—Measures eye movement.
  - Polysomnogram (PSG)—Combines of the findings of the EEG, EMG, and EOG.
- Insomnia
  - Description—Trouble initiating sleep, has frequent awakenings, ineffectual sleep (not refreshed) episodes, and excessive daytime sleepiness.
- Narcolepsy
  - Description—Client suddenly falls asleep or has sudden hallucinations.
  - Leads to uncontrollable need for sleep and may cause a sudden loss of muscle tone, which can lead to accidents.
- Sleep apnea
  - Description—Client experiences no breath 10 seconds or longer; is observed in obese clients and those who use alcohol or tobacco or maybe both
  - Is related to or could be a signal of an other illness, pharynx alteration, tonsillar obstruction, nasal obstruction.
  - Leads to hypertension, stroke, pulmonary hypertension, polycythemia.

Important nursing implications	Abnormal findings
Common clinical findings	Patient teaching

OBTAINING HEALTH INFORMATION

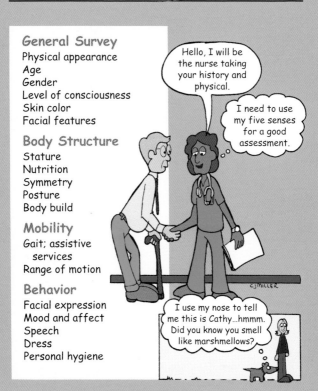

General Survey
Physical appearance
Age
Gender
Level of consciousness
Skin color
Facial features

Body Structure
Stature
Nutrition
Symmetry
Posture
Body build

Mobility
Gait; assistive
  services
Range of motion

Behavior
Facial expression
Mood and affect
Speech
Dress
Personal hygiene

Assessment at a Glance
Obtaining Health Information

- General survey
  - Physical appearance—Does it match with what might be expected for the client's age and sex? Do variations exist that might be explained by socio-cultural factors or that might give clues to underlying disease?
  - Level of consciousness (LOC)—Observation and direct questioning.
  - Other features like skin color and variations, as well as facial features, will also provide valuable information.
- Body structure
  - Stature, position, and posture—Are they consistent with what might be expected? Do deviations exist that may signal psychologic or physiologic needs (slumped shoulders, kyphosis)?
  - Nutrition variations may be obvious if signs of malnutrition or obesity exist.
  - Symmetry, body build, and contour—Facial and body features offer a good guide for "normal." If something is questioned on one side of the body (facial droop, bump on the wrist), then compare it with the other side of the body. Are the extremities held in the same way? Are motions similar on both sides? Are muscles the same size and contour on both sides?
- Mobility
  - Gait and range of motion (ROM)—Are movements smooth and effortless?
  - Variations may be detected with simple unplanned interactions (health interview) or may only be observed during the performance of activities of daily living (ADLs) or musculoskeletal assessment.
- Behavior
  - Facial expression, mood, and affect—Does the appearance of the client's face match the mood that is expected, based on assessment findings? If the client is smiling, would the nurse expect this response at this time? Does the client change expression during conversation?
  - Speech—Is it appropriate? Slurred? Have any recent changes occurred?
  - Dress and hygiene

| Important nursing implications | Abnormal findings |
| Common clinical findings | Patient teaching |

HEALTH HISTORY

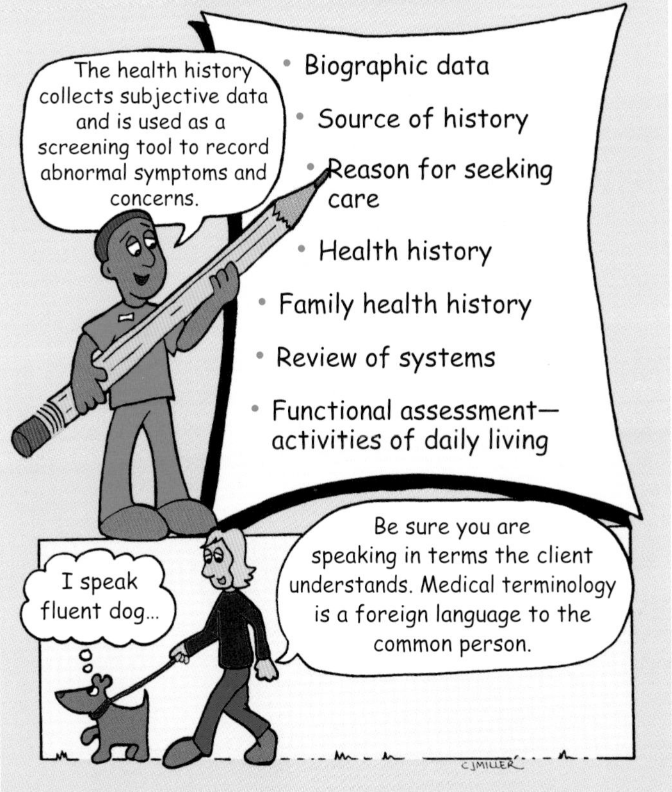

Assessment at a Glance
Health History

KEY CONCEPTS

- Biographic data—Obtain full name, address, occupation, and birth date.
- Source of history—Always attempt to verify data against two sources (client, chart; client, family; family, chart). Be careful not to violate confidentiality standards in the process of verification.
- Reason for seeking care—Nurses need to understand what is most important to the client. Ask the client to describe why they sought care in the first place. Providing attention to the client's main concern will create an alliance that will facilitate success in the health care process.
- Health history—Inquire about previous hospitalizations, surgeries, childhood illnesses, immunizations, allergies, and current medications.
- Family health history—Many health issues can be traced to family characteristics. Family history should include information related to habits, traditions, disease, and attitudes of the family.
- Social history—A client's social interactions can greatly affect his or her health (occupation requiring lots of typing, sitting, breathing in of chemicals). Education may be correlated with the client's ability to understand instructions. Significant others can be either a threat or an asset to the success of the care plan.
- Review of systems—Evaluate each body system as described by client.
- Functional assessment—Evaluate the client's performance of ADLs and instrumental ADLs (IADLs) and his or her self-care ability.
- "Medicalese"—Avoid using medical terms that may confuse and frustrate the client. Use language and terms that are easily understood by the client.

Important nursing implications	Abnormal findings
Common clinical findings	Patient teaching

INTERVIEWING

1 Opening

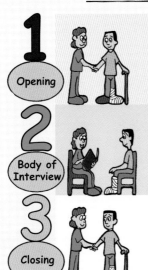

Establishing Rapport...
"Hi, I'm Ashley, and I'll be interviewing you and doing your physical assessment."

2 Body of Interview

Necessary Questions...
Age, gender, marital status, occupation, religion, allergies, reason for visit, treatments, medications, history, family history, surgeries, health habits...

3 Closing

Closing the Interview...
"That is all I need right now. Thank you for your time. Do you have any questions?"

The quality of the interview is based on your communication skills to help you gather credible information and to establish a therapeutic relationship with your client.

Gotta go, gotta go!

==================== **Assessment at a Glance** ====================
Interviewing

Interviews are important for data collection and for building a therapeutic relationship with the client.
- Environment
  - Privacy is a must.
  - Comfort—Does the client need to be in a gown through the entire interview? Will he or she be cold?
  - Equal status seating—Keep an open area between you and the client; maintaining eye level with the client is preferable.
  - Distractions—Television, family, or pain may distract the client.
  - Refuse interruptions—Have another nurse monitor your calls. Telephone calls should be restricted.
- Opening
  - Establishing a team approach—"I am going to collect information that will allow you and I to come up with your plan of care."
  - Giving permission to interrupt—"Please stop me if you have a question."
  - Teaching—The nurse should look for teaching opportunities throughout the interaction.
- Body of the interview
  - Open-ended questions—best for exploration
  - Closed questions—when specific clarification is needed
  - Note taking—acceptable but not to the point that the client thinks the notes, computer, or chart is more important than he or she is
  - Nonverbal communication—The nurse should look to the client's nonverbal mannerisms to verify and validate the information being gathered.
- Closing
  - Reflection and interpretation—Review what is being conveyed.
  - Validate observations.

Important nursing implications	Abnormal findings
Common clinical findings	Patient teaching

SUBJECTIVE VS. OBJECTIVE

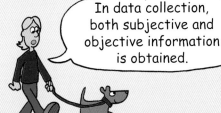

SUBJECTIVE	OBJECTIVE
Verbal information evident only to the client	Information obtained through the senses and hands-on examination

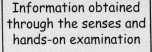

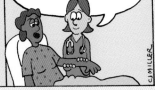

==
Assessment at a Glance
Subjective vs. Objective
==

SUBJECTIVE DATA

- Evident only to the source; from client, family member, or friend
- Usually involves feelings, emotions, and perceptions
- Amount of medication taken; when certain events occurred

OBJECTIVE DATA

- Obtained through the senses of the nurse; vital signs and other measurements
- Lung and heart sounds, range of motion, appearance, observations

SUBJECTIVE AND OBJECTIVE DATA

- Pain—May be subjective in nature, but the nurse will need to quantify pain ratings, quality, radiation, cause, and relieving factors. These data will be considered objective in certain venues because pain is continually tracked for changes.
- Chart—Data from the client's chart are usually considered objective, but consider that some of the reports contain subjective information.
- Reports—Other health care providers will offer information and is usually considered objective but will need to be verified with other objective findings.

VALIDATION

- The nurse should strive to verify assessment findings with other findings (client reports shortness of breath on exertion, crackles are heard in the right base, the x-ray study shows infiltrates in the right base).
- Whenever possible, findings should be validated with the client for clarification, teaching, and developing a therapeutic relationship.

Important nursing implications	Abnormal findings
Common clinical findings	Patient teaching

SIGNS AND SYMPTOMS

A symptom is a subjective sensation described by the client.

A sign is an objective abnormality that the examiner detects on physical examination.

"I feel like I have to pee all the time."

"It burns and feels like I'm peeing razor blades."

"I just ache all over."

Abdominal Tenderness
- Cloudy urine
- Increased temperature
- Fever and chills
- Increased voiding
- Laboratory values showing increased white blood cell count and increased bacteria

When you put together the signs and symptoms, the client's condition becomes more clear.

Hmmm!

Assessment at a Glance
Signs and Symptoms

DEFINITION OF SYMPTOMS

- Subjective findings are reported by the client.
- May be expressed in ways different than what the nurse is expecting (ache, discomfort, movement, buzzing, weird feeling).
- Confusion can also make symptom description, detection, and assessment difficult to interpret, and a caregiver for the client may need to assist in interpreting nonsensical comments or actions.

SYMPTOMS

- Place the client's words in quotes.
- Assess for
  P (provocative and palliative)
  Q (quality and quantity)
  R (region and radiation)
  S (severity scale)
  T (timing and onset)
  U (understanding client perceptions)

DEFINITION OF SIGNS

- Objective abnormalities are detected by the examiner.
- May be response to an intervention, observation of body fluids, assessment findings, and results of diagnostic testing.

SIGNS

- Identify symptom, connect sign.
- Symptoms give important clues to guide physical assessment.
- Use professional terms, and describe signs completely.

| Important nursing implications | Abnormal findings |
| Common clinical findings | Patient teaching |

GORDON'S 11 FUNCTIONAL HEALTH PATTERNS

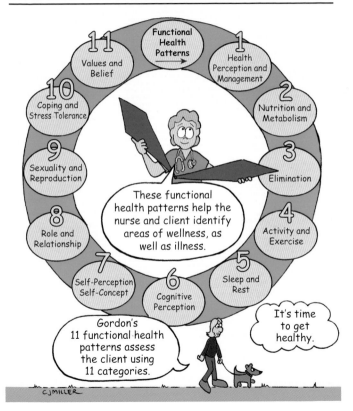

==
Assessment at a Glance
Gordon's 11 Functional Health Patterns
==

Gordon's 11 functional health patterns can serve as a systematic approach to health assessment.

KEY CONCEPTS

- All 11 functional health patterns need to be addressed in certain situations or focused visits.
- Data can be categorized in multiple areas.
- Search for subjective and objective signs and symptoms in all areas.

11 FUNCTIONAL HEALTH PATTERNS (EXAMPLES)

- Health perception and management—practices and perceptions related to health, wellness, quality of life
- Nutrition and metabolism—practices, perceptions, family effects, socioeconomic effects; cultural, ethnic, religious practices
- Elimination—bowel, bladder, integument; effects on self-concept
- Activity and exercise—limitations in activities of daily living (ADLs), compensation for limitations, effects on socialization, safety
- Sleep and rest—patterns, employment considerations, recent changes
- Cognitive perception—alertness, orientation, self-management, safety, caregiver in the client's life, educational background
- Self-perception and self-concept—psychologic issues and mental health, recent changes in behavior, "What do others think about you?"
- Role and relationship—significant other, client's responsibilities to others, safety, cultural characteristics
- Sexuality and reproduction—family history, significant others, health education issues, safety
- Coping and stress tolerance—commonly used coping mechanisms, physical signs of persistent stress
- Values and beliefs—social circles, faith practices and beliefs, alternative medicines and therapies

Important nursing implications	Abnormal findings
Common clinical findings	Patient teaching

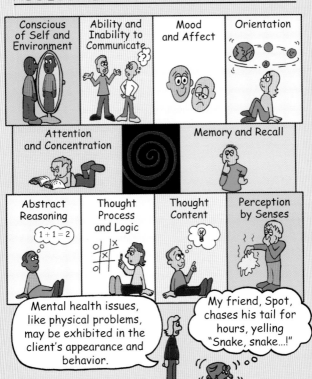

==
Assessment at a Glance
Assessment of Mental Status
==

KEY CONCEPTS

- Prioritize the mental health and physiologic health needs based on Maslow's "Hierarchy of Needs."
  - Physiologic—physical survival
  - Safety and security
  - Social belonging
  - Self-esteem
  - Self-actualization
- ADPIE (acronym for **a**ssessment, **d**iagnosis, **p**lanning, **i**mplementation, **e**valuation)—The nursing process is just as effective when providing mental health nursing care as with other types of nursing care.
  - Numerous tools exist to assist in mental health assessment: McMaster Family Assessment Device, Hamilton Anxiety Scale, Mania Rating Scale, Mini-Mental State Examination

MENTAL HEALTH ASSESSMENT AREAS

- Consciousness—alert, safety, able to navigate in the world around them
- Language—communication issues
- Mood and affect—emotional expressions and manifestations
- Orientation—perception of time and space
- Attention—ability to concentrate, stay on task, safety
- Memory—short term, long term
- Abstract reasoning—comprehension of ideas such as caring, thankfulness
- Thought processes—ability to make sense of issues and rationalize
- Thought content—obsessions, topics, issues
- Perceptions—awareness of reality, including hallucinations, delusions, illusions, paranoia

Important nursing implications	Abnormal findings
Common clinical findings	Patient teaching

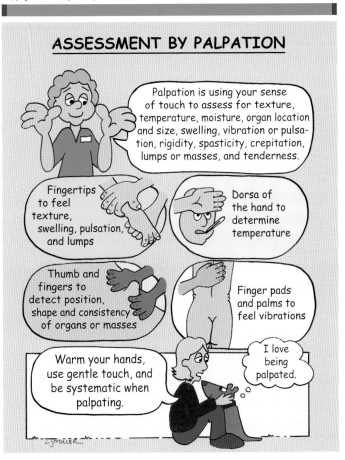

============ Assessment at a Glance ============
Assessment by Palpation

KEY CONCEPTS

- Palpation follows inspection.
- Wash hands. Gloves can prevent the detection of important information. Use critical thinking to assess the risk or need for gloves (open areas, infestations, or infections on the nurse's hands or the client's body). Standard Precautions should always be maintained.
- Warm hands. Perform light-to-deep palpation (least invasive to most invasive).
- Do not ignore the client while palpating.
- Use subjective information to identify and confirm the need for palpation.
- Palpate painful areas last. Observe the client's face when palpating.
- Compare sides for symmetry.
- Perform hand hygiene after palpation.

PALPATION TECHNIQUES

- Fingertips—Texture, swelling, raised area, pulsation, lumps. May alternate fingertips to verify assessment. Avoid confusing your pulse with the pulse of the client. Crepitus is like crunching cereal and may be associated with joint disease or air trapped in subcutaneous tissue (pneumothorax).
- Thumb and finger grasp—Position, shape, consistency, size, mobility of organs or masses. May need to use other techniques to assist in confirming observations. Nodules under the skin can be secured with thumb and finger and then moved by a kneading action with three fingers.
- Dorsa of hand—When assessing temperature variations, compare both sides.
- Vibrations—Are best detected with the fingers (usually the base) and the ulnar side of the hand.
- Abdomen should be percussed and ausculated before palpation.
- OB—Cup hand to check fundus.

| Important nursing implications | Abnormal findings |
| Common clinical findings | Patient teaching |

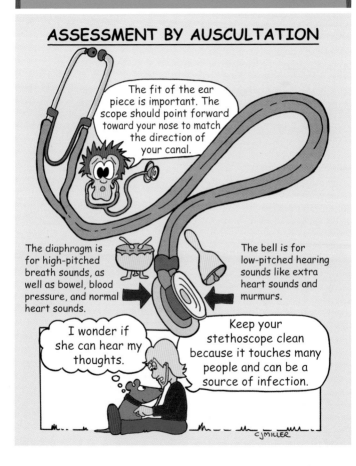

Assessment at a Glance
Assessment by Auscultation

KEY CONCEPTS

- Stethoscopes
  - If sounds are not heard well, then determine whether the bell or diaphragm is on and the earpieces are pointed forward.

TECHNIQUE

- No matter what body system, create a preferred pattern technique and use it on all clients. A consistent pattern decreases the chances of missing an area. Examples might include:
  - APTM (**a**ortic, **p**ulmonic, **t**ricuspid, and **m**itral) regions for cardiovascular auscultation
  - Clockwise pattern for abdominal auscultation
- Auscultate before palpations or interventions—Palpating may alter the sounds heard in a particular area.
- Push firmly enough to observe a light circle on the skin when the stethoscope diaphragm or bell is removed. If pushed lighter, then too many extra noises will be heard; if pushed harder, then the sound may be altered.
- Diaphragm-only stethoscope—High-end stethoscopes with only a diaphragm becomes a bell with low pressure and a diaphragm with hard pressure.
- Control the tubes of the stethoscope to prevent bumping.
- Palpate only one carotid artery or radial pulse when listening to heart tones.
- Ask the child to blow at a tissue to enhance breath sounds.
- Avoid listening over clothes, gowns, or sheets unless in an emergency situation.

ENVIRONMENT

- Turn down the television.
- Ask family members to leave.

Important nursing implications	Abnormal findings
Common clinical findings	Patient teaching

ASSESSMENT OF THE PULSE

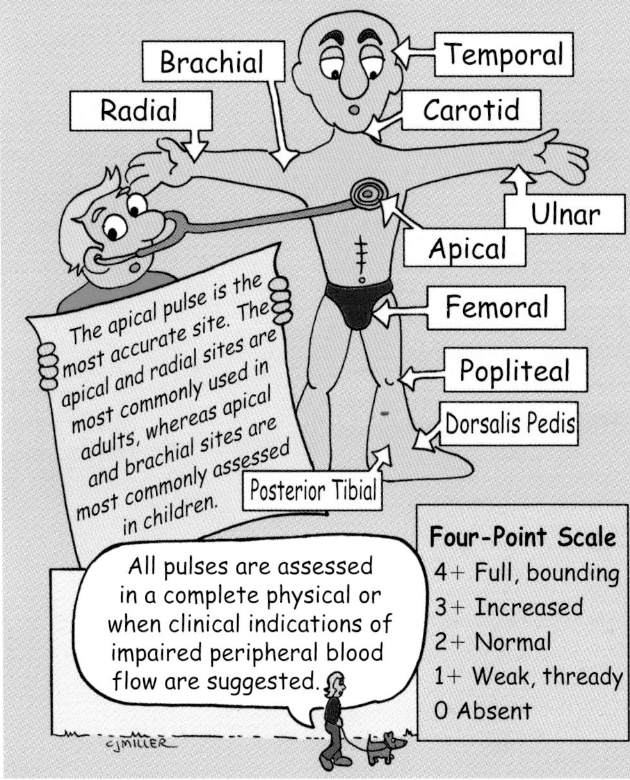

Brachial

Temporal

Radial

Carotid

Ulnar

Apical

Femoral

Popliteal

Dorsalis Pedis

Posterior Tibial

The apical pulse is the most accurate site. The apical and radial sites are most commonly used in adults, whereas apical and brachial sites are most commonly assessed in children.

All pulses are assessed in a complete physical or when clinical indications of impaired peripheral blood flow are suggested.

Four-Point Scale
4+ Full, bounding
3+ Increased
2+ Normal
1+ Weak, thready
0 Absent

CJMILLER

Assessment at a Glance
Assessment of the Pulse

NORMAL RANGE OF FINDINGS

- Inspect hair, skin color and texture, and extremity size. Compare symmetry between the right and left sides; symmetry is a sign that pulse quality is equal but may not be necessarily adequate.
- Palpate using the pads of the fingers.
  - Do not count the pulse felt in your own fingertips.
  - Pressing too hard or too soft can lead to an inaccurate count.
  - Carotid pulse should correlate with the S_1 heard in the heart.
  - Do not palpate both carotid arteries at the same time to avoid causing a vasovagal reaction.
- Rate—Count for 1 full minute to identify irregularities.
  - Adults: 60 to 100 beats per minute (bpm) (lower in athletes); children: 70 to 120 bpm; infants: 70 to 190 bpm
- Rhythm—Should be the same rhythm felt the entire time.
- Force—+2 is considered "normal"; some clients may be normal at +3 or +1.
  - Feet have a slightly weaker force than the radial and carotid arteries.
- Infants—Vital signs should be taken with the least invasive method.
- Pregnancy can increase the heart rate 15 to 20 bpm.

ABNORMAL FINDINGS

- Inspection—Hair is absent; skin is thin, fragile, or discolored; extremities are atrophied, asymmetric, or swollen.
- Heart rate
  - Tachycardia can be a sign of fever, hypoxia, or anemia. Bradycardia can be a sign of ischemia of the SA node, increased ICP, and vagal stimulation.
- Rhythm—Detection of missed or skipped beats should be noted.
- Force—A 3- or 4-point scale may be used.
  - Inability to detect a pulse may constitute a medical emergency.
  - Doppler ultrasonography should be used to verify the absence of a pulse.

| Important nursing implications | Abnormal findings |
| Common clinical findings | Patient teaching |

ASSESSMENT OF BLOOD PRESSURE

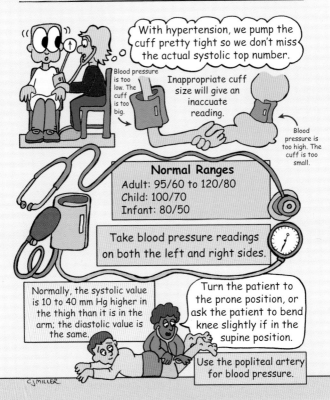

With hypertension, we pump the cuff pretty tight so we don't miss the actual systolic top number.

Blood pressure is too low. The cuff is too big.

Inappropriate cuff size will give an inaccuate reading.

Blood pressure is too high. The cuff is too small.

Normal Ranges
Adult: 95/60 to 120/80
Child: 100/70
Infant: 80/50

Take blood pressure readings on both the left and right sides.

Normally, the systolic value is 10 to 40 mm Hg higher in the thigh than it is in the arm; the diastolic value is the same.

Turn the patient to the prone position, or ask the patient to bend knee slightly if in the supine position.

Use the popliteal artery for blood pressure.

CJ MILLER

--- Assessment at a Glance ---
Assessment of Blood Pressure

EQUIPMENT
- Sphygmomanometer
  - Cuff bladder width is approximately 40% of the extremity circumference.
- Diaphragm of stethoscope
  - Cannot hear? Properly place cuff; elevate arm over head for 1 minute (nurse may hold it up, if needed); lower arm and take BP reading
- Doppler ultrasonography—Use if stethoscope cannot detect sounds.
- Automated machine
  - Invasive BP—Intravenous (IV) cannula is inserted in the radial or femoral artery; sensitive equipment directly measures BP.
  - Noninvasive BP—Cuff is connected to a machine that automatically assesses BP in timed intervals without the use of a stethoscope or Doppler ultrasound.

TECHNIQUE (MANUAL)
- Client rests for 5 minutes before taking a BP reading.
- Bare the arm, and maintain level with the heart.
- Cuff is inflated 1 inch over the brachial artery; medial antecubital fossa.
- Palpate brachial or radial pulses; inflate cuff until pulse is no longer felt (20 to 30 mm Hg beyond feeling pulse to avoid the auscultatory gap).
- Deflate cuff, and wait 1 minute.
- Place the stethoscope over medial antecubital fossa.
- Inflate cuff to 20 to 30 mm Hg from where a pulse is no longer palpable.
- Deflate cuff 2 mm Hg per heart beat.
- Note when sound is first heard (Korotkoff I) and when it is last heard (Korotkoff V).
- Repeat the procedure with the other arm as indicated.
- Teaching—Avoid assessing BP on arms with shunts, with PICC lines, or after mastectomy or after IV infusions.

| Important nursing implications | Abnormal findings |
| Common clinical findings | Patient teaching |

ASSESSMENT OF ORTHOSTATIC (POSTURAL) HYPOTENSION

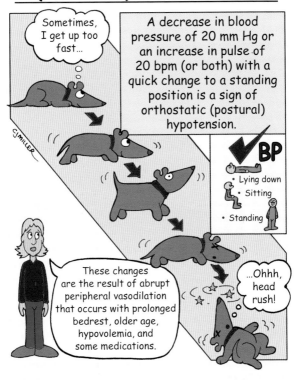

Assessment at a Glance
Assessment of Orthostatic (Postural) Hypotension

Clients who report feelings of lightheadedness, dizziness, fainting, or feeling weak when they sit up or stand should be evaluated for orthostatic (postural) hypotension. As a result of hypovolemia, dehydration, older age, or medication interactions, cardiac output becomes inadequate to perfuse the brain.

EQUIPMENT

- Sphygmomanometer or automated machine
- Cuff bladder width of approximately 40% of the extremity circumference
- Stethoscope

TECHNIQUE

- Client rests for 5 minutes in the lying position before BP reading is taken.
- Bare the arm, and level it with the heart.
- Inflate cuff 1 inch over the brachial artery; medial antecubital fossa.
- Take pulse rate and auscultatory BP (or machine) with the client lying down.
- Record findings, deflate cuff, leave cuff on the arm, and have client sit up.
- Note any symptoms, and provide for safety. Wait 1 minute.
- Take pulse rate and auscultatory BP (or machine) with client sitting up.
- Record findings, deflate cuff, leave cuff on the arm, and have client stand.
- Note any symptoms, and provide for safety. Wait 1 minute.
- Take pulse rate and auscultatory BP (or machine) with client standing.
- Record findings, deflate cuff, and have client sit down.

NORMAL RANGE OF FINDINGS

- No significant change in BP or pulse rate with position change
- No signs or symptoms with position changes

ABNORMAL FINDINGS

- BP decrease of 20 mm Hg or pulse rate increase of 20 beats per minute (bpm)
- Dizziness, lightheadedness, or syncope

Important nursing implications	Abnormal findings
Common clinical findings	Patient teaching

ASSESSMENT OF THE SKIN

1. Skin history?

2. Pigmentation or skin color changes?

3. Problems with blemishes, moles, or sores?

4. Skin dryness, excess moisture, or increased temperature?

5. Pruritis (itch skin)?

6. Abnormal bruising?

7. History of rashes or lesions?

8. Medications?

9. Occupational or environmental hazards?

10. Type of skin care?

Assessment at a Glance
Assessment of the Skin

NORMAL RANGE OF FINDINGS: INSPECT, THEN PALPATE

- Color
  - Palms, plantar surfaces, lips, and oral mucosa tend to be lighter.
- Temperature, texture, moisture
  - Even temperature levels are throughout with some cooling in the extremities.
  - Smooth and firm with the exception of joints and palmar or plantar surfaces where roughness may occur.
  - Skin is dry unless normal perspiration is occurring.
  - Oral and nasal mucosa remain moist.
- Mobility and turgor, thickness
  - Freely movable; no tenting
  - Uniform throughout with some callous and thickening over joints
- Wound healing
  - Inflammation, hemostasis, proliferation, remodeling
  - Closure in several days, complete healing usually within a month

ABNORMAL FINDINGS

- Color
  - Jaundice, pallor, or erythema is present.
  - Variations may be seen in the palm or plantar surface or in the conjunctiva or oral mucosa of dark-skinned individuals.
- Temperature, texture, moisture
  - Hypothermia, hyperthermia; asymmetry between areas
  - Rough, dry, flaky; overly damp, boggy
- Mobility and turgor, thickness, edema
  - Taut, shiny, tenting; fragile, thin, shiny (atrophic)
  - +1 minimal to +4 severe (pitting and nonpitting); weeping
- Lesions
  - Primary or secondary; pattern or grouping; distribution on body

---

Important nursing implications	Abnormal findings
Common clinical findings	Patient teaching

ASSESSMENT OF SKIN FUNCTIONS

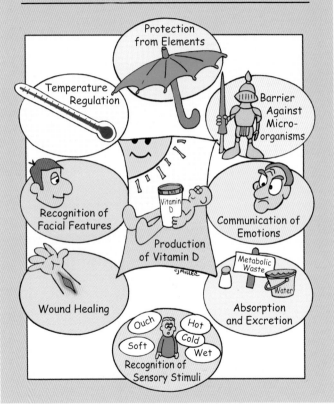

Protection from Elements

Temperature Regulation

Barrier Against Micro-organisms

Recognition of Facial Features

Production of Vitamin D

Vitamin D

Communication of Emotions

Metabolic Waste

Water

Wound Healing

Absorption and Excretion

Ouch   Hot

Soft   Cold   Wet

Recognition of Sensory Stimuli

Assessment at a Glance
Assessment of Skin Functions

NORMAL RANGE OF FINDINGS

- Protection
  - Intact skin can prevent loss of moisture to the environment.
  - Can repel water, as well as cold and hot air to a certain extent.
  - Holds in adipose tissue that can serve as insulation.
  - Normal flora keeps troublesome organisms from causing infection (yeast).
- Communication
  - Gives shape to the muscles underneath.
  - Emotions are often communicated by manipulating the muscles underneath (frown, smile, pout).
- Absorption, secretion, and metabolic
  - Offers a way for chemicals to enter the environment (urea, NaCl).
  - Odor is present.
  - When ultraviolet rays strike the skin, vitamin D is synthesized.
- Sensory
  - Skin has many sensors that send information (hot, cold, sharp, dull, stretch) to the brain.
  - Hair on the skin is very sensitive to movement.
- Thermoregulation
  - Vasodilation may bring blood closer to the skin surface to enable heat to dissipate; warm, erythematous skin.
  - Vasoconstriction may keep blood from the surface to maintain the core temperature; skin may be lighter in color and is usually cooler.
  - Sweat evaporates off the skin when heat is transferred from the body to the atmosphere.

Important nursing implications	Abnormal findings
Common clinical findings	Patient teaching

ASSESSMENT OF THE HAIR

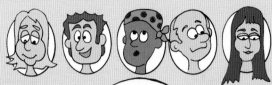

Questions to Ask in Assessment:

- Have you had changes in hair texture?
- Have you had hair loss (alopecia)?
- Was it sudden or gradual?

Hair Loss Causes:

- Heredity?
- Chemotherapy?
- Toxic alopecia?
- Seborrheic dermatitis?
- Tinea capitis (ringworm)?
- Pediculosis (head lice)?
- Folliculosis?

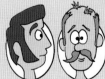

Assessment at a Glance
Assessment of the Hair

NORMAL RANGE OF FINDINGS

- Subjective
  - Have changes in hair quality and pattern occurred?
  - Were the changes sudden or gradual?
  - Are changes correlated with life events (pregnancy)?
- Color
  - Black to light blonde
  - Graying varies, depending on genetics (usually after 30 years of age)
- Distribution
  - Normal patterns for the individual, gender, age
- Quantity, thickness, texture
  - Some areas may have less hair than in other places; is genetically determined; is soft or coarse; curly, straight, or kinky.

ABNORMAL FINDINGS

- Color
  - Missing pigmentation, dyes; premature graying
- Distribution, quantity, thickness, texture
  - Hirsutism (too much or undesired)—Facial hair in women
  - Alopecia (loss)—Causes include male-pattern balding, chemotherapy, injury, infection (tinea)
  - Course and dry (hypothyroidism) or straight and shiny (hyperthyroidism)
  - Head lice (tinea capitis), pubic lice (tinea pubis)

| Important nursing implications | Abnormal findings |
| Common clinical findings | Patient teaching |

ASSESSMENT OF THE NAILS

Splinter hemorrhage—
Reddish brown or dark
streaks under the nail caused
by bacteria or trauma

Koilonychia (spoon nails)—
Thin nails with edges turned
up; may be hereditary, congenital,
or indicate iron deficiency

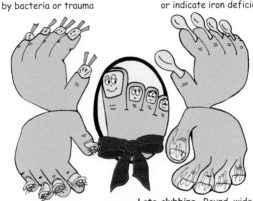

Onycholysis—Thickened, brittle,
dark nails as a result of fungal
invasion

Late clubbing—Round, wide fingertips
seen with chronic obstructive
pulmonary disease, congestive heart
disease, and cyanosis

Nail care is
very important.
I get regular
"pet"-icures.

In assessing nails, ask
whether the client has
experienced any changes
in the quality of their nails.
When did they first notice
the change?

Assessment at a Glance
Assessment of the Nails

NORMAL RANGE OF FINDINGS

- Subjective
  - Ask about changes in color, consistency, and shape.
  - Ask about self-care practices and footwear.
- Shape and contour—Usually smooth and slightly rounded.
  - Borders approximated; skin is without erythema, edema, and exudate.
  - Angle of nail to nail bed is approximately 160 degrees.
- Consistency
  - Firm yet pliable; adheres to the nail bed with firm palpation.
- Color—Pink undertone (may be darker in individuals with darker skin).
  - Few white streaks from incidental injury may be observed.

ABNORMAL FINDINGS

- Shape and contour
  - Koilonychia (spoon nails)—Thin nails with edges turned up; hereditary, congenital, iron deficiency anemia.
  - Clubbing—Rounded nails that are slightly spongy with a nail bed angle of 180 degrees; may indicate chronic hypoxia.
  - Thickened and ridged nails indicate arterial insufficiency.
  - Jagged edges may be related to trauma or biting.
- Consistency
  - Spongy or thickened
  - Onycholysis—thickened brittle and dark color—result of fungal infections
- Color
  - Dark, bluish-purple, yellowing
  - Splinter hemorrhage—reddish brown dark streaks, related to bacterial infections (may indicate subacute bacterial endocarditis)
  - Brown linear streaks (may indicate melanoma)
  - Cyanotic nail beds (indicates hypoxia)

| Important nursing implications | Abnormal findings |
| Common clinical findings | Patient teaching |

ASSESSMENT OF THE HEAD

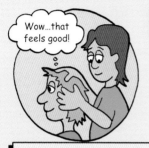

Questions to Ask

- Do you have headaches or tender areas?
- Can you describe any changes in your hair or skin?
- Do you have any teeth or vision problems?
- Is there any discharge from your nose or ears?

Things to Check

- Symmetry
- Size related to body
- Facial structures and features
- Jaw movement
- Swelling
- Muscle twitching
- Eye movement
- Skin quality and pigmentation

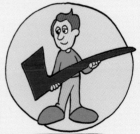

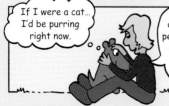

=== **Assessment at a Glance** ===
Assessment of the Head

SUBJECTIVE

- Headaches, tenderness, paresthesias, twitching, trouble eating or swallowing
- Change in hair and skin, lesions, oronasal discharge
- Variations that are not normal for the client

OBJECTIVE: INSPECT, THEN PALPATE

- Shape, contour, and size
  - Side-to-side comparison
  - Symmetry of size and position ("Is this variation normally this way for you?")
  - Normocephalic, atraumatic
- Hair and skin
  - Pattern, distribution, texture, color
- Musculoskeletal system
  - Free of uncontrolled movements
  - Free jaw movements without crepitation
- Vasculature
  - No abnormal bulging, pulsations, thrills, or bruits
- Infants and children
  - Head circumference should be measured each visit until 2 years of age.
  - Newborn—Head circumference is 2 cm less than the chest circumference.
  - Two-year-old child—Head circumference is equal to the chest circumference.
  - Fontanels are smooth and mostly flat (no bulging or sunken areas).
  - Posterior fontanel—1 cm diameter at birth and closes in 1 to 2 months.
  - Anterior fontanel—May be nonpalpable at birth and closes between 9 and 24 months.

Important nursing implications	Abnormal findings
Common clinical findings	Patient teaching

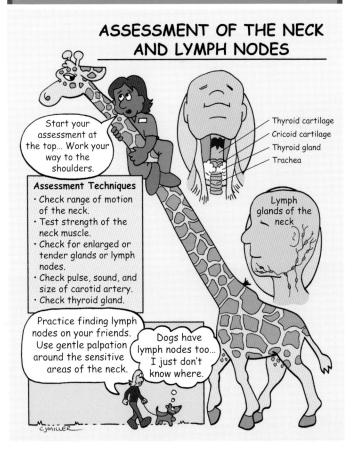

ASSESSMENT OF THE NECK AND LYMPH NODES

Start your assessment at the top... Work your way to the shoulders.

Thyroid cartilage
Cricoid cartilage
Thyroid gland
Trachea

Lymph glands of the neck

Assessment Techniques
- Check range of motion of the neck.
- Test strength of the neck muscle.
- Check for enlarged or tender glands or lymph nodes.
- Check pulse, sound, and size of carotid artery.
- Check thyroid gland.

Practice finding lymph nodes on your friends. Use gentle palpation around the sensitive areas of the neck.

Dogs have lymph nodes too... I just don't know where.

Assessment at a Glance
Assessment of the Neck and Lymph Nodes

NORMAL RANGE OF FINDINGS

- Subjective
  - Headaches, difficulty moving, pain with movement
  - Lumps, masses, swallowing, breathing, vertigo
  - History of injury or surgery; occupational hazards
  - Thyroid—current medications, weight loss or gain, mood changes, hair changes, thermoregulation
- Inspection
  - Symmetry—Head centered; thyroid and accessory muscles symmetrical.
  - Pulsations—May be visible anterior to the sternomastoid (bilaterally right to left) when client as supine at 45 degrees.
  - Trachea—Is midline; thyroid rises smoothly or symmetrically over trachea; no masses or unilateral enlargement
- Auscultation
  - Bell; medial edge of sternomastoid muscle on both sides. Ask client to hold his or her breath while the nurse holds his or her own breath; slight hum may be normal; bruits, swishing, murmurs may be observed.
- Palpation
  - Carotid pulse—Palpate one side at a time.
  - Trachea—Is symmetrically centered.
  - Thyroid—Feel for lobe of the thyroid to glide under the fingers; nontender, barely palpable if at all.
  - Cervical chain lymph nodes—Nurse's fingerpads applies gentle kneading in small circles with gentle pressure; client's head tilts forward.
  - Pick a pattern—Do not vary sequence.
  - Range of motion (ROM) against resistance
- ROM and strength
  - Active ROM then against resistance

Important nursing implications	Abnormal findings
Common clinical findings	Patient teaching

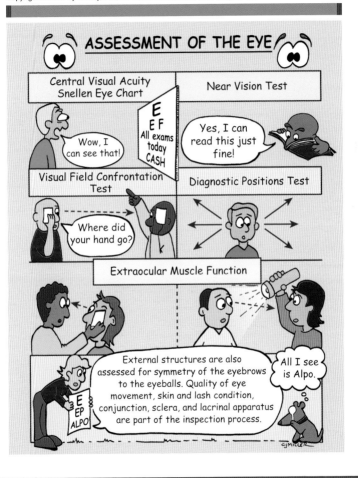

Assessment at a Glance
Assessment of the Eye

NORMAL RANGE OF FINDINGS

- Visual acuity
  - Snellen—20 feet, corrected and uncorrected
  - Near vision (Jaeger card)—14 inches from eye or client reads from a magazine or newspaper
- Inspection
  - Symmetry—canthus, position on face
  - Iris, pupil, sclera, cornea—lesions (lids covers upper one third of the iris)
  - Sunken, protruding (exophthalmos)
  - Eyebrows, lashes—distribution, lesions, quantity
  - Cover test—Ask client to stare at your nose, cover one eye, and watch uncovered eye for abnormal movement.
  - Peripheral fields—Conduct confrontation test: 2 feet nose-to-nose, cover opposite eye (nurse's left and client's right).
  - Accommodation—Look far (mydriasis), then look near (nurse's finger is 3 inches from nose). Assess pupillary constriction and convergence of eyes.
  - Corneal light reflex—Shine penlight directly at nose from 12 inches.
  - Red reflex—Shine penlight into eye. Should see orange-red.
  - Pupillary light reflex—Darken room and ask client to look far. Advance light from side to assess constriction of pupil (mydriasis). Evaluate simultaneous constriction of other pupil—consensual light reflex.
  - PERRLA—**P**upils are **E**qually **R**ound and **R**eactive to **L**ight and **A**ccommodation.
- Palpation
  - Blink reflex—When the cornea and lashes of one eye are touched, both eyes blink.

| Important nursing implications | Abnormal findings |
| Common clinical findings | Patient teaching |

ASSESSMENT OF THE EAR

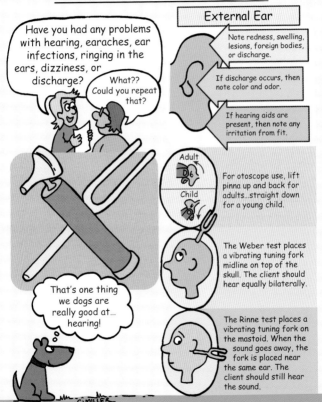

Assessment at a Glance
Assessment of the Ear

NORMAL RANGE OF FINDINGS

- Auditory acuity
  - Hearing test (whisper)—1 to 2 feet
  - Bone conduction (BC) and air conduction (AC)
  - Weber—Place tuning fork stem on top and center of skull. "Where do you hear this best?" Sound should be bilaterally equal.
  - Rinne—Time this assessment. Instruct client to say, "Now" when no sound is heard.
    - Activate the tuning fork, place stem on mastoid process (BC).
    - When the client says, "Now," place the tuning fork about 2 inches from the outside of the same ear (BC).
    - Normal is a positive Rinne test; AC is greater than BC.
- Inspection
  - Symmetry—Position on the head; top of the auricle lines up with the corner of the eye.
  - Otoscopic evaluation—Pull pinna up; pull back for adults.
  - Insert otoscope slowly, observing integrity of the auditory canal, foreign bodies, and cerumen (light to dark brown).
  - Canal points to the client's nose.
  - Tympanic membrane is intact, pearly gray. The umbo and manubrium are visible; cone of light points toward the chin.
- Palpation—Is firm, nontender, and free of warmth.
  - Tug pinna up and down; tragus.
  - Mastoid process—No tenderness or pain is observed.
- Infants and children
  - Infants should startle with loud sound that is out of sight.
  - Otoscopic examination—Pull pinna straight down.

| Important nursing implications | Abnormal findings |
| Common clinical findings | Patient teaching |

ASSESSMENT OF THE NOSE

Do you suffer from nasal discharge, frequent colds, nose bleeds, sinus pain, or allergies; or have you had trauma to your nose?

I think I'm allergic to cats!

Assessment Tools

Otoscope

Use the otoscope with a short, wide-tipped nasal speculum and a flashlight. Look for external skin problems of the nose, nostrils, and midline in relationship to the face. Palpate for pain. Check nostril patency and nasal cavities.

The Nose

Check the nostrils for moisture, smoothness, tissue color, deviation of septum, swelling, lesions, discharge, foreign bodies, or bleeding.

Press your thumbs over the frontal sinuses (wait... not on the eyeballs, but over the eyebrows!) and on the maxillary sinuses below the cheekbones using a careful firm pressure.

CJMILLER

Does that hurt?

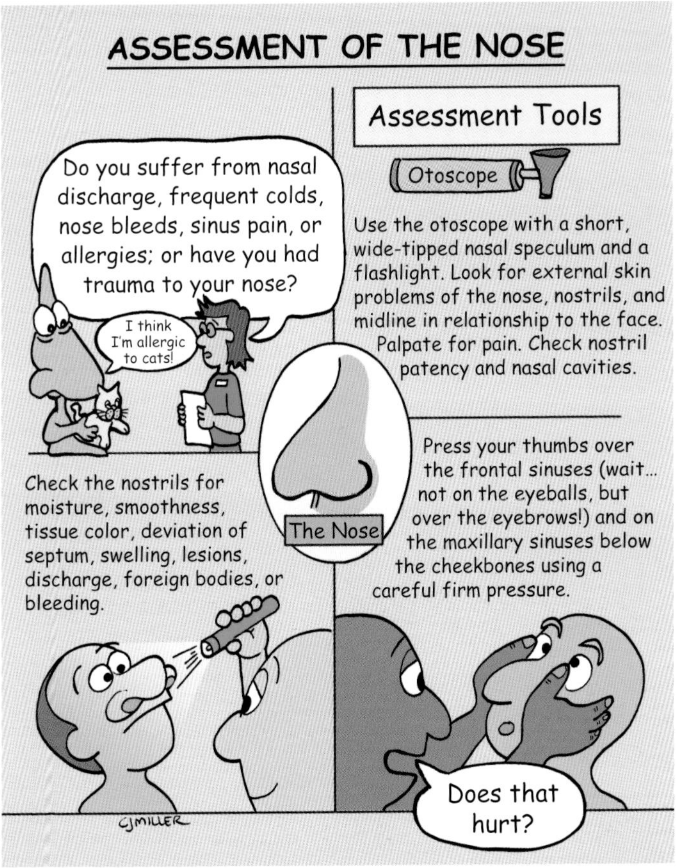

===== Assessment at a Glance =====
Assessment of the Nose

NORMAL RANGE OF FINDINGS

- Smell assessment
  - Use an aromatic (coffee) and fragrant scent (vanilla extract).
  - Test both nares.
- Inspection
  - Symmetry—Position on face; maintain nasal bridge symmetry.
  - Inspect intact skin around nares; look for discharge.
  - Otoscopic evaluation—Use nasal speculum cover; may also use the flashlight and a metal nasal speculum tool.
    - Lift tip of the nose, tilt head back.
    - Insert speculum slowly, observe integrity of the septum. Are mucous membranes intact? Examine for polyps, discharge, and foreign bodies.
    - Light pink is normal.
    - Remember that the nasal cavity goes straight back and NOT up.
  - Palpation—Is firm, nontender; assess for patency by blocking one nare.
- Sinuses—Assess frontal and maxillary.
- Infants and children
  - Nasal patency is important in newborn infants because they breathe through the nose (have suction ready).
  - Nasal ridge is flat in Asian and African-American children.
  - Do not use the metal nasal speculum tool on infants and small children.
- Pregnancy
  - Congestion and epistaxis may be more prevalent as a result of increased vascularity of the upper respiratory system.
- Older adult
  - Nose becomes more prominent, and nasal hair becomes more coarse.
  - Smell decreases with age.

Important nursing implications	Abnormal findings
Common clinical findings	Patient teaching

ASSESSMENT OF THE MOUTH AND THROAT—QUESTIONS

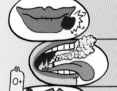 Do you get mouth sores?

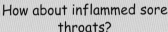 How about inflamed sore throats?

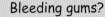 Bleeding gums?

 Do you have sensitive teeth or get toothaches?

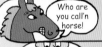 Do you have hoarseness or voice changes?

 Any problems swallowing (dysphagia)?

 Do you have a bad taste or an alteration in your taste?

 Do you smoke? Do you drink? How often?

Assessment at a Glance
Assessment of the Mouth and Throat—Questions

- Sores and lesions—gingival, mouth, tongue
  - Locations (particular area, multiple spots)? How many (clustered, single)?
  - What makes it better (medications, temperatures, foods, textures)?
  - What makes it worse (situations, stress, temperatures, foods, textures)?
  - Frequency (monthly, just in winter, after a trip, examination week)?
  - Significant others with similar issues?
- Inflamed throat
  - Issues with allergies or postnasal drip?
  - Habits (drug abuse, alcohol use, tobacco use)?
  - Medical treatments (radiation to the neck)? Frequency, onset, duration?
  - What makes it better or worse? Previous streptococcal infections?
  - Correlation with humidity or time of day?
- Bleeding gums
  - Last dentist appointment? Dental hygiene (brushing and flossing)?
  - Medications (anticoagulants)? Frequency, onset, duration?
- Teeth sensitivities and aches
  - Related to hot or cold? Tooth loss?
  - Most recent dental visit? Dental hygiene practices?
- Hoarseness
  - Feeling of lump or pain in the throat? Frequency, onset, duration?
  - What makes it better or worse? Correlation with humidity or time of day?
  - Others with this issue? Associated with another illness?
  - Use of voice in hobby or vocation?
- Swallowing difficulties
  - Medical history of pneumonia, stroke, gastroesophageal reflux disease (GERD), cancer? Pain?
- Taste
  - Change in smell? Continuous or intermittent problem?
  - Correlated to life events (cancer, pregnancy, stress issue)?
- Alcohol and tobacco use

Important nursing implications	Abnormal findings
Common clinical findings	Patient teaching

ASSESSMENT OF THE MOUTH AND THROAT

Check the internal and external surfaces of the lips for moisture, color, cracks, and sores.

Look at the color, and feel the gums for swelling, lesions, bleeding, and moisture. Check the teeth for damage, looseness, and appropriate number.

Observe the tongue for texture, color, moisture, sores, and overall appearance. Check the U-shaped area under the tongue for growth or lesions.

Check the buccal mucosa for growths, color, moisture, and possible skin tags from the molars biting the inside of the ckeek.

Palpate the throat while checking for lumps or soreness on one side at a time.

Check the color of both the anterior hard palate and the soft palate.

Check uvula for color, location, and size.

Check tonsils for the size and color. Is blood present? Check the gag reflex (cranial nerves IX and X).

CJMILLER

Assessment at a Glance

Assessment of the Mouth and Throat

NORMAL RANGE OF FINDINGS

- Inspection
  - Use penlight, clean gloves; use gauze and tongue blades to move tongue for visualization and for gag reflex.
  - Symmetry—mouth position on face, shape of mouth and neck
  - Skin around mouth intact, chelitis, cracking, discharge, moisture, color
  - Mucosa pink, moist, lesions; skin tags, molar biting
  - Gingiva, moist, pink lesions, approximation to teeth
  - Teeth caries, intact, missing, gingival borders, coloration; bite pattern
  - Tongue texture, moist, pink, growths or lesions, ventral surface vascularity, lesions, frenulum intact
  - Hard and soft palates, light pink, intact, no openings or lesions
  - Soft palate and uvula rise with phonation (rise is symmetric and smooth), is moist
  - Tonsils, tonsillar pillars—size, exudate, light pink
- Palpation—firm, nontender
  - Gingiva firm, swelling, mass, tenderness
  - Tongue firm, lesions, mass
  - Throat—external, nontender, no mass or lesions
  - Gag reflex bilaterally with stimulation (cranial nerves [CN] IX and X)

ABNORMAL FINDINGS

- Inspection
  - Smile is uneven, unable to puff cheeks.
  - Cherry red lips may indicate poisoning or acidosis; blue lips may indicate cyanosis or hypothermia; pallor suggests anemia.
  - Fruity or foul breath exists—diabetes or liver failure.
  - Beefy red or glossy tongue is observed—pernicious anemia.

Important nursing implications	Abnormal findings
Common clinical findings	Patient teaching

ASSESSMENT OF THE BREAST

- Be considerate and concise when assessing.
- Palpate axilla area to check for lumps, tenderness, swelling, or rashes.
- Assess breasts for pain, symmetry, lumps, or thickness.
- Discharge?
- History of trauma?
- Are monthly self-examinations done?
- Are annual physical examinations with regular mammograms done?

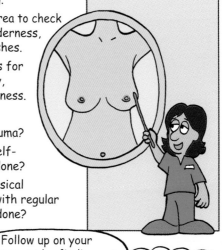

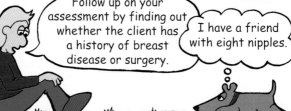

Follow up on your assessment by finding out whether the client has a history of breast disease or surgery.

I have a friend with eight nipples.

Assessment at a Glance
Assessment of the Breast

INTERVIEWING

- Attempt to conduct as much of the interview with the client fully dressed (warmth, dignity). However, opportune teaching times will occur during the physical examination
- Medical history—Includes menarche, pregnancies, births, abortions (spontaneous or other).
- Family history is important, especially when related to breast cancer.
- General structure—Includes symmetry and supernumerary nipples.
- Pain? Does monthly cycle make it better or worse?
- Discharge? Occurs cyclical? Similar to pregnancy?
- Color, consistency, odor; lumps; tenderness; swelling
- Trauma (accidental, abuse, surgery); yeast or thrush, particularly with nursing
- Nursing—history with children
- Frequency of breast self-examination (BSE)? Annual physical with mammogram?

DURING PREGNANCY

- BSE is still important.
- Breasts enlarge starting in the second month of gestation.
- Nipples and areola enlarge and become darker.

OLDER ADULT

- Loss of glandular and adipose tissues causes the breasts to be flattened and hang down in the later decades of life.
- Mammograms and BSE are still important.

MALE BREAST

- Gynecomastia is common in the male adolescent; will spontaneously resolve.
- Gynecomastia is common in the older male adult when testosterone levels decrease. Male BSE is recommended.

Important nursing implications	Abnormal findings
Common clinical findings	Patient teaching

BREAST EXAMINATION

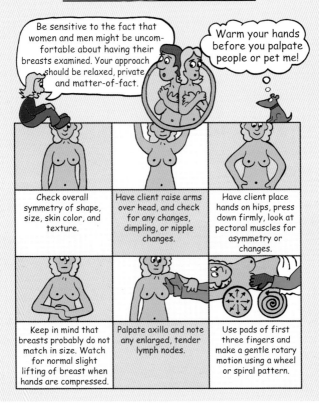

Be sensitive to the fact that women and men might be uncomfortable about having their breasts examined. Your approach should be relaxed, private, and matter-of-fact.

Warm your hands before you palpate people or pet me!

Check overall symmetry of shape, size, skin color, and texture.	Have client raise arms over head, and check for any changes, dimpling, or nipple changes.	Have client place hands on hips, press down firmly, look at pectoral muscles for asymmetry or changes.
Keep in mind that breasts probably do not match in size. Watch for normal slight lifting of breast when hands are compressed.	Palpate axilla and note any enlarged, tender lymph nodes.	Use pads of first three fingers and make a gentle rotary motion using a wheel or spiral pattern.

Assessment at a Glance
Breast Examination

NORMAL RANGE OF FINDINGS

- Inspection—Keep the client covered and as comfortable as possible (warm room and hands).
- Client should be involved. "Is this normal or a new change?"
- Neutral position—Place arms at the side with the client sitting.
  - Note general symmetry, size, shape.
  - Observe skin texture throughout (color, blemishes, redness).
  - Note dimples or lumps; examine supraclavicular or axillary areas for swelling or discoloration. Note nipple direction, discharge, or lesions.
- (1) Arms are raised above the head → (2) Hands on hips and press up → (3) Press hands together in front of abdomen → (4) Nurse holds client's hands, and client leans forward for breast inspection.
  - Position change of the breasts
  - Symmetric movement and free forward movement
  - Dimpling or retractions with position change
  - Accentuation of skin texture
  - Nipple direction change

PALPATION—USE WARM HANDS

- Axilla—Hold client's left arm with nurse's left hand.
  - With right hand in left axilla, massage with finger pads in a diamond shape (center of humerus and bicep to fifth lateral intercostal space, tail of Spence to scapula).
  - Look for swelling, tenderness, or nodes in this area.
- Breast and tail of Spence—Client is lying on back with rolled towel under the shoulder of the breast being examined.
  - Pick a pattern (spokes of a wheel or spiral) and stick to it.
  - Press two to three fingers firmly enough to identify mass or tenderness.
- Nipple—Client is lying on the back; attempt to express discharge.

| Important nursing implications | Abnormal findings |
| Common clinical findings | Patient teaching |

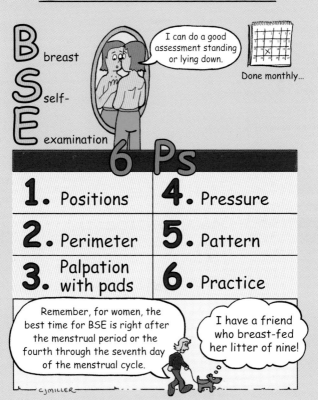

===== Assessment at a Glance =====
Breast Self-Examination

The client should know that the annual examination is not adequate alone for breast health screening.

6 Ps OF BSE

- Positions
  - Standing—Looking in a mirror, raise hands over head, hang arms by side, place hands on hip and push up, place hands together and push.
    - Look for changes in shape, contour, size, and asymmetry.
  - Lying—Lie on back or side for palpation. Raise arm over head on side being assessed.
    - Use right hand to assess left and right breasts.
  - Side-lying or leaning forward—Allows women with pendulous breasts to better assess all areas.
- Perimeter
  - Collarbone (clavicle)—Examine middle of armpit down to below the lower border of the breast (midaxillary) and middle of the breastbone up to the clavicle.
  - Most cancers develop in the upper outer region (tail of Spence).
- Palpation with finger pads
  - Use two to three finger pads (circles the size of dimes).
  - Cover all areas thoroughly; do not lift fingers from skin between areas.
- Pressure
  - Apply light-to-deep pressure to cover all layers of the breast.
- Pattern
  - Spokes of the wheel; spiral out
  - Palpate in vertical strips and tissue under nipple
  - Pinch nipple gently in two directions; look for discharge.
- Practice
  - Perform at least one side in front of a practitioner at the annual examination to ensure proper technique.

Important nursing implications	Abnormal findings
Common clinical findings	Patient teaching

ASSESSMENT OF THE THORAX AND LUNGS
(INSPECTION OF THE POSTERIOR CHEST)

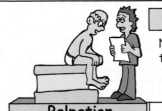

Inspection

Note the posture that the client assumes for optimal breathing.

Palpation

Move from top to bottom symmetrically to assess symmetrical chest expansion.

Tactile Fremitus: The client says "99" while the nurse feels the vibration.

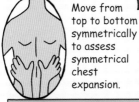

Percussion

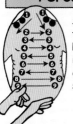

Start at the apices. Percuss interspaces, comparing side to side.

Auscultation

Use the diaphragm of the stethoscope, progressing from side-to-side comparison.

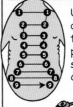

Assessment at a Glance
**Assessment of the Thorax and Lungs
(Inspection of the Posterior Chest)**

NORMAL RANGE OF FINDINGS

- Inspection—Keep the client covered and as comfortable as possible (warm room, hands, and stethoscope).
  - Landmarks—C7, T12, costal vertebral angle, scapula (no auscultation or percussion over scapula)
  - Anatomy—three lobes on right, two lobes on left, diaphragm at T10 on exhalation and T12 on inhalation
  - Posture—symmetrical movement
- Palpation—Use warm hands.
  - Symmetrical chest expansion—Wrap hands around the bottom of the rib cage; thumbs should barely touch.
  - Tactile fremitus—Use the pads of the fingers or the ulnar side of the hand; client says "99"; palpate apex to base, compare side-to-side.
- Percussion
  - Percuss interspaces, apex to base, compare side-to-side.
- Auscultation—Use warm stethoscope.
  - Diaphragm, compare side to side.
- Infants and children
  - Ask the child to blow on a tissue to accentuate breath sounds.
  - It is acceptable to listen to an infant's lungs while the infant is crying. The deep breath between cries can help hear adventitious sounds.
  - Apgar score should be 7 to 10 at birth.

Important nursing implications	Abnormal findings
Common clinical findings	Patient teaching

ASSESSMENT OF THE THORAX AND LUNGS
(INSPECTION OF THE ANTERIOR CHEST)

Assess and palpate. Look for symmetry, shape, and configuration of the chest.

Ask the client to take a deep breath. Watch and feel, using your thumbs and fingers. Adjust to the movement.

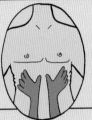

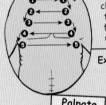

Percussion sequence: Have the client say "99" while you feel the vibration. Then percuss from the top, working your way down from side to side.

Expected (Normal) Sounds

Liver: dullness
Stomach: tympany
Cardiac: dullness
Muscle and bone: flat
Between ribs: resonance

Palpate

Percuss

Auscultate

The things I do for attention!

Although it seems like a lot of information to balance, we expect normal findings... Watch and listen for the abnormal.

CJ MILLER

—————————— **Assessment at a Glance** ——————————
Assessment of the Thorax and Lungs
(Inspection of the Anterior Chest)

NORMAL RANGE OF FINDINGS

- Inspection—Keep the client covered and as comfortable as possible (warm room, hands, and stethoscope); usually requires gown to be placed on lap for this assessment. May be able to cover the back with a gown or blanket during anterior thoracic assessment.
- Landmarks—sternal notch, angle of Louis, supraclavicular notch, costal angle and margin

SYMMETRICAL MOVEMENT

- Transverse to anteroposterior diameter (2:1); does not include breasts or adipose tissue.

SPECIAL SITUATIONS

- In an emergency, the anterior chest may be assessed alone; otherwise, the posterior area should always be assessed as well.

ABNORMAL FINDINGS

- Inspection
  - Tripod position (chronic obstructive pulmonary disease)
  - Retractions or bulging in the interspaces
  - Use of accessory muscles (airway obstruction, atelectasis)
  - Barrel chest (transverse to anteroposterior diameter of 1:1)
- Palpation—Use warm hands.
  - Asymmetrical chest expansion
  - Tactile fremitus—increased or decreased vibration (consolidation)
- Percussion—dull or flat or hyperresonant
- Auscultation—crackles, wheeze, diminished or absent breath sounds

Important nursing implications	Abnormal findings
Common clinical findings	Patient teaching

ASSESSMENT OF THE HEART
(AREAS AND DESCRIPTIONS)

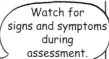

Watch for signs and symptoms during assessment.

I ♥ my heart.

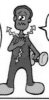

I feel like an elephant is sitting on my chest.

- Pain or tightness
- Numbness and tingling
- Dull or sharp pain
- Is chest pain relieved by nitroglycerin?

Chest Pain (Angina) or Related Cardiac Symptoms

I feel so short of breath!

- Orthopnea (need to be upright to breathe)
- Cyanosis or pallor

Dyspnea (Shortness of Breath)

I'm coughing so hard that I keep waiting for my lungs to come out!

- Fluid in lungs
- Inability to perform activities of daily living without fatigue

Cough (Productive or Nonproductive Fatigue)

Seems like I need to get up a lot at night to pee!

- Needs to get up at night to void
- Edema in extremities

Edema and Nocturia

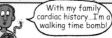

With my family cardiac history...I'm a walking time bomb!

- Cardiac history
- Sedentary lifestyle
- Poor diet
- Smoking
- Excessive alcohol intake
- Medications

Personal Family History and Personal Health Habits

Assessment at a Glance

**Assessment of the Heart
(Areas and Descriptions)**

SUBJECTIVE DATA

- Chest pain
  - Need to consider onset, duration, quality, location, radiation (jaw or left arm), intensity, and rating.
  - What makes it worse or better? Does it go away after ingesting an antacid? Do medications have an effect (nitroglycerin)?
  - Have you felt this type of pain before?
  - Does the pain change with external manipulation (push on muscles)?
  - Pain presentation in women can be different than it is in men (nausea).
  - Is it associated with diaphoresis, nausea, and palpitations?
- Dyspnea
  - Is it associated with any exercise? If so, how much and what type of exercise (dyspnea on exertion [DOE])?
  - Is there pain at rest? Is it intermittent or constant? Does it wake the client?
- Orthopnea
  - Do you sleep in a recliner? How many pillows do you need to sleep?
- Cough
  - Productive or nonproductive (color, odor, blood-tinged)?
  - Associated with peripheral edema?
- Fatigue
  - Unusual? Sudden or gradual onset? Able to perform activities of daily living?
- Cyanosis or pallor
  - Does it come and go? Is it associated with an activity or event?
- Edema
  - Dependent? Jugular venous distension? When does it occur the most?
- Nocturia
  - Are you up frequently at night? Does edema develop during the day?
- Medical history, family history, personal habits

Important nursing implications	Abnormal findings
Common clinical findings	Patient teaching

ASSESSMENT OF THE HEART AND VASCULAR NECK

Anatomy and physiology are the keys to pathophysiology.

I wonder if my tail wags to the beat of my heart.

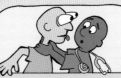

When palpating the carotid arteries...keep in mind that they provide blood flow to the brain. **Palpate one side at a time.**

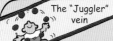

The "Juggler" vein

The jugular is for upper body venous return. Watch for bulging because it is a sign of fluid overload and right-sided heart failure.

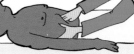

Pressure under the rib cage at the liver forces extra blood to drain from the liver, causing a temporary bulge in the jugular vein.

The apical pulse is located at the fourth or fifth intercostal space between the medial and midclavicular line.

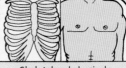

Skeletal and physical landmarks aid in stethoscope placement when listening for heart sounds.

<hr/>

Assessment at a Glance

Assessment of the Heart and Vascular Neck

NORMAL RANGE OF FINDINGS

- Inspection
  - Precordium—heaves, lifts, bulging, pulsations
  - Neck—bulging or pulsations
  - Landmarks—sternal notch, angle of Louis, second intercostal space (ICS), fifth ICS, midclavicular line (MCL), anterior axillary line
- Palpation—Use warm hands.
  - Apical impulse—fifth ICS, left MCL; pad of one finger (lateral deviation; could indicate cardiomegaly)
  - Unpalpable in approximately one half of adults
  - Client lies on left side to accentuate impulse.
  - Use palm of the hand—Palpate the left sternal border, heart apex, and base for any pulsations or thrills.
  - Palpate carotid pulse one side at a time, using two fingers from the middle of neck medial to the sternomastoid muscle.
- Auscultation—Use warm stethoscope.
  - APTM areas of the heart—Listen in the **a**ortic, **p**ulmonic, **t**ricuspid, and **m**itral regions. (Think of mnemonic to help remember sequence—**ap**e **t**o **m**an.)
  - May need to palpate pulse while listening to identify S_1 and S_2 heart sounds.
  - Always try to find S_1 and S_2 heart sounds in all four areas.
  - Listen to the apical pulse (apex—fifth ICS and left MCL) for 60 seconds.
  - Note rate and rhythm.
  - Palpate carotid pulse while listening to apical pulse. S_1 heart sound should correlate with the carotid pulse.

<hr/>

Important nursing implications	Abnormal findings
Common clinical findings	Patient teaching

ASSESSMENT OF HEART SOUNDS— HARMONY OF THE HEART

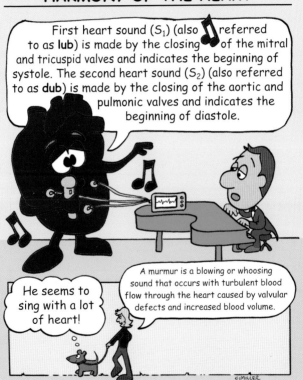

First heart sound (S$_1$) (also referred to as **lub**) is made by the closing of the mitral and tricuspid valves and indicates the beginning of systole. The second heart sound (S$_2$) (also referred to as **dub**) is made by the closing of the aortic and pulmonic valves and indicates the beginning of diastole.

A murmur is a blowing or whoosing sound that occurs with turbulent blood flow through the heart caused by valvular defects and increased blood volume.

He seems to sing with a lot of heart!

===== Assessment at a Glance =====
Assessment of Heart Sounds—Harmony of the Heart

NORMAL SOUNDS

- Lub-dup (S_1 and S_2)
  - S_1 (lub) is heard best at the apex. S_2 (dup) is heard best at the base.
  - Tricuspid (T) and mitral (M) valves are heard best at the apex.
  - Aortic (A) and pulmonic (P) valves are heard best at the base.
- Systole
  - Begins with S_1 (T and M close); the left ventricle ejects blood into the aorta, and the right ventricle ejects blood into the pulmonary artery.
  - Ends with S_2 (A and P are closed).
  - Pulmonary vein drains into left atrium. Vena cava drains into right atrium.
- Diastole
  - Begins with S_2 (A and P are closed); atria eject blood into the ventricles through the T and M.

MURMURS

- Intensity—Grade I is barely audible through grade VI, which is very loud.
- Innocent—Midsystolic, low-grade murmurs are often benign.
- Location (clue as to which valve may be the origin of the murmur)
  - Base or apex; A, P, T, or M
- Timing (clue as to which valve may be the origin of the murmur)
  - A, P, T, or M stenosis or regurgitation

EXTRA HEART SOUNDS

- Split S_2—Aortic valve is closing sooner that the pulmonic valve.
- S_3—Vibration of ventricular filling during diastole is heard.
  - Occurs with heart failure and volume overload (ventricular gallop).
  - May be normal in children and young adults.
- S_4—Heard in late diastole when ventricular filling is particularly difficult.
  - Occurs with coronary artery disease (CAD), cardiac myopathy, aortic stenosis, increased blood pressure (atrial gallop).
  - May be normal in older adults with no cardiovascular disease after exercise.

ASSESSMENT OF BLOOD VESSELS AND LYMPHATIC SYSTEM—QUESTIONS

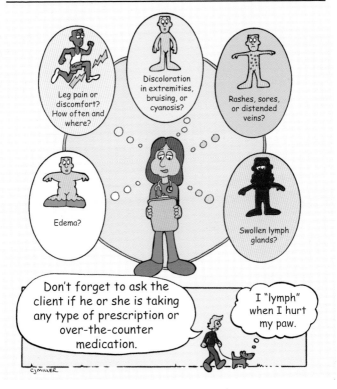

Assessment at a Glance
Assessment of Blood Vessels and Lymphatic System—Questions

MEDICAL HISTORY

- Heart disease, stroke, peripheral vascular disease, venous insufficiency
- Diabetes, chronic wounds (poor wound healing)
- Surgery (mastectomy, coronary artery bypass [CAB], grafts, tonsillectomy)
- Leg pain and discomfort
  - Location, onset, duration, quality, radiation
    - Associated with exercise? Other precipitating factors?
    - What makes it better? Any swelling with the pain?
    - Any hot or cold areas with the pain?
    - Does the pain come with hot or cold environment?
    - Does the pain wake the client at night?
- Discoloration of extremities
  - Redness, pallor, cyanosis or blueness, brown
    - How long has the color change been present (1 hour, 1 day, 1 year)?
    - Has the temperature changed at the site of the discoloration?
    - Has exudate or weeping occurred at the sight of discoloration?
    - Has a change in color occurred with a change in position?
- Lesions on extremities
  - Generalized or localized
    - Have patches developed over certain areas (patterns)?
    - Is it unilateral or bilateral?
    - How long has it been there, and has the lesion changed?
    - Is any exudate or weeping associated with the lesion?
- Swelling, edema, or lymphadenopathy
  - Is swelling constant or intermittent? Associated with a position change?
  - Is swelling associated with weeping (dependent edema)?
  - Is swelling associated with trauma, pain, heat, redness or hardened skin?
  - Is edema near a surgical site (saphenous graft from CAB)?
  - Are swollen nodes only in one area or all over? Nodes unilateral or bilateral?

Important nursing implications	Abnormal findings
Common clinical findings	Patient teaching

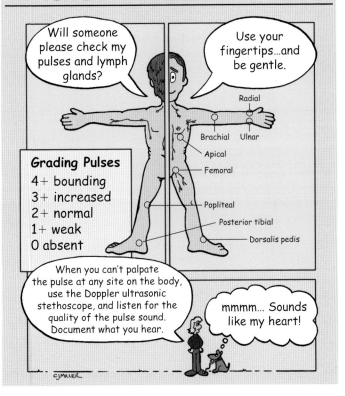

Physical Assessment of Blood Vessels and Lymphatic System

NORMAL RANGE OF FINDINGS

- Diagnostics
  - Is the blood pressure (BP) the same in both arms?
- Inspection
  - Inspect areas of swelling, asymmetry, or lumps.
  - Most pulses are not seen and cannot be heard by the ear alone.
  - Skin is smooth, intact, and free of lesions.
  - Hair patterns on extremities show expected distribution.
  - Scars may require an explanation of variations.
- Palpation—Use warm hands.
  - Warmth—Compare temperature bilaterally with the dorsum of the hands.
  - Apical impulse—fifth intercostal space (ICS), left midclavicular line (MCL); pad of one fingertip (lateral deviation could indicate cardiomegaly)
    - Unpalpable in about one half of adults.
    - Client lies on left side to accentuate pulse.
  - Capillary refill time is less than 3 seconds.
  - Peripheral pulse palpation usually requires two fingers. Do not move the fingers while palpating (i.e., no kneading or massaging).
  - Popliteal pulse—Is difficult to find; it may not be necessary to assess if pedal pulses are adequate.
  - Pedal pulses—A light touch is often necessary to locate these pulses.
  - Femoral pulse—Frog leg position may help expose this area.
  - Carotid pulse—Assess one side at a time.
  - Lymph node palpation—Use a moderate amount of pressure in a kneading or gentle massaging motion.
  - Edema assessment—Pitting or nonpitting; assess by pushing against a bony prominence if possible.
- Auscultation—Doppler ultrasound for nonpalpable pulses; use conducting gel.

| Important nursing implications | Abnormal findings |
| Common clinical findings | Patient teaching |

FIVE Ps OF NEUROVASCULAR ASSESSMENT

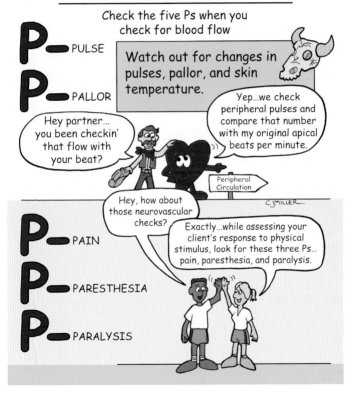

Five Ps of Neurovascular Assessment

The neurovascular assessment is indicated in many situations. The client may have had an injury (motor vehicle accident, burn). The client may have a vascular disease, such as arteriosclerosis, that puts him or her at risk for peripheral vascular disease. Some may also have a clotting or embolic disorder, such as atrial fibrillation or endocarditis, or the client may simply complain of his or her arm, hand, leg, or foot feeling funny.

NORMAL RANGE OF FINDINGS

- Pulse
  - Dorsalis pedis, posterior tibial, radial, capillary refill time (CRT)
  - Compare the quality of the pulse on both extremities. It should be symmetrical in both radial pulses or in both dorsalis pedis pulses.
  - 0 = absent; +1 = weak; +2 = normal; +3 = strong; +4 = bounding
  - CRT <3 seconds
  - Doppler ultrasonography is used if needed.
- Pallor
  - Color of the extremity is the same as the skin elsewhere.
  - No cyanosis, paleness, ruddy, or brawny colorations are observed.
- Pain
  - No pain with rest, activity, or weight bearing. Note pain scale rating.
- Paresthesia
  - No numbness, tingling, burning, or pins and needles reported.
- Paralysis
  - Activity is symmetrical, and strength is strong (5).
    - 5 – against gravity and resistance
    - 4 – against gravity and minimal resistance
    - 3 – against gravity
    - 2 – minimal and not fully against gravity
    - 1 – contraction detected
    - 0 – flaccid

Important nursing implications	Abnormal findings
Common clinical findings	Patient teaching

ASSESSMENT OF THE ABDOMEN— QUESTIONS

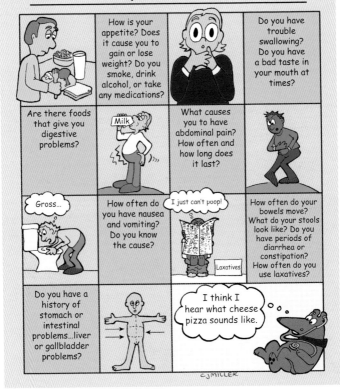

Assessment at a Glance
Assessment of the Abdomen—Questions

MEDICAL HISTORY

- Medications; allergies and food intolerances; tobacco and alcohol use
- Menstrual cycle, pregnancies, sexually transmitted diseases
- Surgeries; appetite (weight loss/gain); psychologic concerns (anorexia, bulimia)
- Pain
  - Location, onset, duration, quality, radiation
    - Associated with meals?
    - Are other precipitating factors (urination, intercourse) present?
    - What makes it better? Any swelling with the pain?
    - Is nausea associated with the pain? Does the pain wake client at night?
    - Does it change with movement or pressure on the abdomen?
- Eating
  - Coughing with eating (dysphagia)? Food getting stuck?
  - Reflux or burning (before, after, or during meals)?
  - Coughing at night? Change in taste?
- Nausea
  - With or without emesis. Associated with eating or smells? Pain?
    - Do sudden movements cause nausea? Describe emesis color and consistency.
    - Timing of nausea and vomiting? What makes the nausea better or worse?
- Bowel habits
  - Abnormalities in the stool or bowel patterns
    - Normal patterns? Discoloration of the stool? Pain with bowel movement?
    - Unusual amounts of flatus? Formed, liquid, explosive? Bloating?
    - Do hydration issues occur? (Older adults are frequently dehydrated.)
- Genitourinary system
  - Issues related with the renal or sex organs
    - Irregular menses? Discharge? Pain with intercourse? Bleeding?
    - Odor to the urine? Discoloration of urine?

Important nursing implications	Abnormal findings
Common clinical findings	Patient teaching

ASSESSMENT OF THE ABDOMEN—
INSPECT AND AUSCULTATE

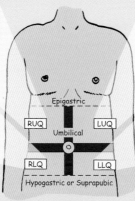

Right Upper Quadrant

Left Upper Quadrant

Right Lower Quadrant

Left Lower Quadrant

Epigastric

RUQ LUQ

Umbilical

RLQ LLQ

Hypogastric or Suprapubic

Sequence of Physical Assessment
1. Inspect abdomen.
2. Auscultate for 1 full minute in each quadrant.
3. Percuss for tympany and dullness.
4. Palpate surface and deep areas.

Practice, practice, practice using your stethoscope. Use it on yourself, your family... even your dog! Become familiar with the sounds of the body.

When my stomach growls...I growl BACK!

CJ MILLER

Assessment at a Glance
Assessment of the Abdomen—Inspect and Auscultate

NORMAL RANGE OF FINDINGS

- Inspection
  - Use tangential lighting—Standing straight on and from the side, note any asymmetry and contours (scaphoid, flat, rounded).
  - Pulsations or movements? Scars, lesions, moles, striae?
  - Demeanor—Guarding? Lying in the fetal position?
  - Tubes (peritoneal dialysis)? Appliances (colostomy or urostomy)?
  - Is skin free of redness, inflammation, and jaundice?
- Auscultation
  - Pick a pattern and stick to it (RUQ, LUQ, LLQ, RLQ—clockwise).
  - Listen in each area (should hear 5 to 30 bowel sounds per minute).
  - Use the diaphragm for bowel sounds.
  - Assess aorta and renal arteries with the bell to identify any bruits.

ABNORMAL FINDINGS

- Inspection
  - Note areas of swelling and asymmetry.
  - Protruding masses (hernia, everted umbilicus)?
  - Reddened area of skin? Jaundice? Ascites?
  - Cutaneous angiomas (high pressure from portal hypertension causes abdominal vasculature to become more visible—spider nevi)?
  - Pulsating mass may indicate an aortic aneurysm or intestinal obstructions.
- Auscultation
  - Tinkling sounds may indicate obstruction.
  - Hyperactive high-pitched sound may indicate obstruction.
  - Hypoactive to absent sounds? (Absent sounds can be an emergency.)
  - Bruits? (Reassess the heart sounds to ensure bruits are not a murmur echo.)

| Important nursing implications | Abnormal findings |
| Common clinical findings | Patient teaching |

ASSESSMENT OF THE ABDOMEN—PERCUSS AND PALPATE

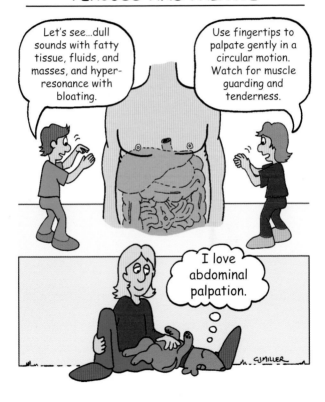

Assessment at a Glance
Assessment of the Abdomen—Percuss and Palpate

Stress and tension could make percussion and palpation not only uncomfortable for the client but also change the assessment findings (tense abdominal muscles). Encourage client to voice concerns.

PREPARATION
- Empty bladder (urine sample if needed); ensure warm hands and room.
- Client assumes supine position, head on pillow, and knees elevated (less tension on the abdominal wall).

NORMAL RANGE OF FINDINGS
- Percussion
  - Generalized tympany with dullness over the liver and spleen
  - Dull sounds with fatty tissue, fluids, masses
  - Hyperresonance with bloating
- Palpation—Normal liver span 6 to 12 cm (adult)
  - Should include light and deep palpation. (Remember to watch the client's face for signs of discomfort.)
    - 1 inch for light massaging action
    - 2 to 3 inches for deep action (May need both hands.)
    - Assess painful areas last.
    - If the client is ticklish, then place his or her hand under yours.
- Liver palpation
  - Patient takes a deep breath; as they are exhaling, press in with the right hand. Is nontender and usually not palpable.

ABNORMAL FINDINGS
- Percussion
  - Dullness or hyperresonance can indicate a pathologic condition.
- Palpation
  - Note masses or pockets of fluid. Liver border is very prominent.
  - Client is guarded and does not allow the nurse to assess a certain area.
  - Rebound tenderness could indicate peritonitis or appendicitis.

ASSESSMENT OF THE MUSCULOSKELETAL SYSTEM—QUESTIONS

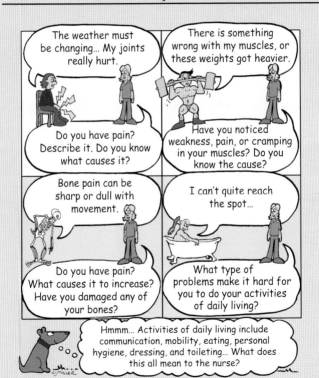

======== Assessment at a Glance ========
Assessment of the Musculoskeletal System—Questions

HISTORY

- Injuries and trauma (frequent patterns such as wrist or hip fractures)
- Occupational hazards (repetitive motions, heavy lifting, bending, squatting)
- Hobbies (sky diving, knitting, woodworking)
- Sleeping surface and positions (new bed) affecting how the client feels
- Surgeries (orthopedic or trauma repair), physical therapy, or chiropractic care
- Diagnostic tests (magnetic resonance imaging [MRI], computed tomographic [CT] scanning), which may remind the client of an issue otherwise forgotten
- Family history of osteoporosis, cancer
- Smoking
- Dietary consumption (calcium and vitamin D)
- History of blood clots, diabetes, cellulitis
- Alternative treatments (biofeedback, herbal medications)
- Pain: Location, onset, duration, quality, and radiation
  - Associated with movement? Other precipitating factors?
  - What makes it better? Any swelling with the pain?
  - Any warmth or coolness or change in color in the area of the pain?
  - Does pain wake the client at night? Stiffness in what areas?
  - Does it change with movement or pressure on the affected area?
  - Stiffness associated with a time of day or activity (or lack thereof)?
- External observations
  - What the client sees on the outside of the body
    - Erythema, ecchymosis, edema? Lesions, deformity?
- Movement—Limited range of motion?
  - Recent changes in movement (weakness, gait disturbance)? Stumbling?
  - Change in posture, sleeping position? Exercise regimen?
  - Activities of daily living—changes in recent abilities to care for self?
  - Recent weight changes?

Important nursing implications	Abnormal findings
Common clinical findings	Patient teaching

ASSESSMENT OF THE MUSCULOSKELETAL SYSTEM—PHYSICAL ASSESSMENT

Check joints of the body for size, color, swelling, masses, or deformities.

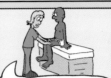

Check the quality of the skin, temperature, and joint areas for abnormalities like tenderness and swelling.

Demonstrate active range of motion for various joints. Use gentle, passive range-of-motion exercises to show limitations.

Have the client push or pull against resistance. Assess for joint movement, muscle appearance, strength, and tenderness.

Assessing a client's musculo-skeletal issues should begin when you first see the client. Observing his or her movements during your introduction will allow you to assess mobility needs.

My normal movements include daily walks!

Assessment of the Musculoskeletal System—Physical Assessment

NORMAL RANGE OF FINDINGS

- Inspection
  - Gait, posture, mobility; no tremors, fine motor muscles intact and smooth
  - Joint size and shape; skin color, texture, lesions; edema
- Palpation
  - No warmth; no masses under the skin or in the muscle or joint space.
  - No crepitus, clunking, crunching, or tenderness with palpation.
- Range of motion (ROM)
  - Freely mobile in expected directions.
  - No instability, pain, paresthesias, numbness, or limitations.
- Strength—Create a pattern to avoid missing areas.
  - Against gravity and resistance; opposing muscle groups (bicep and triceps)
  - Abduction and adduction of joints; observe for balance and proprioception.
  - Use rating scale (5, 4, 3, 2, 1, 0) with range of 5–normal contractions to 0–no contractions against resistance.

ABNORMAL FINDINGS

- Inspection
  - Altered posture, tremors (intentional or at rest); signs of anxiety, pain
  - Joint size (swelling), shape (deformity), lesions, color, mobility
  - Erythema, ecchymosis
  - Scoliosis (When the client bends at the waist, is one shoulder blade higher than the other?); kyphosis
- Palpation
  - Warmth; masses (under the skin, in the muscle or joint space)
  - Crepitus, clunking, crunching; tenderness with palpation
- ROM
  - Limited or altered ROM, instability; pain, paresthesias, numbness, limitations
- Strength—Create a pattern to avoid missing certain areas.
  - Limited movement or flaccidity; loss of balance

ASSESSMENT OF MALE GENITALIA— QUESTIONS

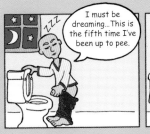

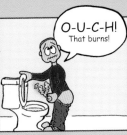

- Do you urinate during the night? How often?
- Do you have a feeling of urgency or pain before, during, or after you urinate?
- Can you describe any problems you are having when you urinate?
- Do you strain to start or to maintain your stream?
- Do you dribble after you leave the restroom or when you sneeze?

- Do you have discolored urine...dark, bloody, no color?
- Is urination painful?
- Is there any discharge from your penis?
- Are you sexually active? Have you ever had any urinary infections or sexually transmitted diseases?
- Do you have multiple sex partners?
- Do you use protective barriers or contraceptives?
- Have you had any surgeries related to your male urinary system?

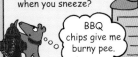

===== Assessment at a Glance =====
Assessment of Male Genitalia—Questions

HISTORY

- Injuries and trauma
- Sexual satisfaction, activity, and practices; oral or anal sex practices; sexually transmitted diseases
- Birth—migratory testes or cryptorchidism; childhood—mumps (orchitis)
- Family history—prostate or testicular cancer
- Genitourinary, renal, or reproductive disease or surgery (varicocele, vasectomy)
- Testicular self-examination practices
- Structure and lesions
  - Relating to the penis and testes
    - Erythema or ecchymosis? Swelling or bulging?
    - Changes associated with straining or lifting?
    - Testes hang freely? Masses or nodules?
    - Lesions, blisters, ulcers, chancre? Exudate? Infestations?
    - Erections adequate, inadequate, or prolonged?
    - Foreskin moves freely; any associated exudate, erythema, or lesions under the foreskin?
- Urinary pattern and characteristics
  - Careful questioning is important because these symptoms can be hard to describe.
    - Frequent voidings of small amounts?
    - Urgency to void?
    - Urgency after voiding? Incontinence? Hesitancy to begin stream?
    - Decreased force of stream? Straining to start or maintain stream?
    - Dribbling before or after voiding or with sneezing?
  - Urine color, odor, consistency, clarity (dark, foul, cloudy, red)?
  - Any discharge, pus, oozing?
- Pain
  - Location, onset, duration, quality, radiation

Important nursing implications	Abnormal findings
Common clinical findings	Patient teaching

ASSESSMENT OF MALE GENITALIA

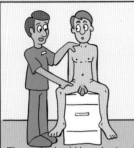

The penis should have horizontal wrinkles around the shaft without blemishes or lesions and the appearance of a dorsal vein.

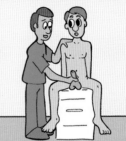

Gently palpate the shaft, and squeeze the glans penis between the finger and thumb.

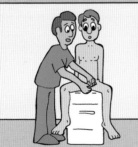

Gently palpate each half of the scrotum for content. Use careful, moderate pressure.

Retract the foreskin on uncircumcised men, or ask the client to do it. Check for cheesy smegma build up under the foreskin. The foreskin must be retracted to its natural position after inspection.

It's just a guy thing...

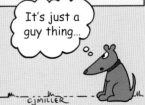

cjMILLER

======= **Assessment at a Glance** =======
Assessment of Male Genitalia

The client should be standing for the examination if possible. Female examiners may wish to have an assistant present for observation.

NORMAL RANGE OF FINDINGS

- Inspection
  - Testes and scrotum freely move, moderate asymmetry
  - Scrotal size varies with temperature changes
  - Multiple wrinkles in the scrotum and circumference of the penis shaft
  - Uncircumcised—foreskin covering the glans, smooth with wrinkled skin at the meatus
  - Circumcised—wrinkled collection of skin at the base of the glans
  - Glans (Foreskin is retracted if needed; be sure to replace.)—lighter color than shaft of penis, smooth, meatus slightly ventral
  - No exudate or buildup under the foreskin
- Palpation
  - Apply gentle, moderately firm pressure between the finger and thumb.
  - Assess shaft of penis for tenderness, masses, and lesions.
  - Glans is soft and pliable.
  - Meatus freely opens with no tissue holding it closed.
  - Check scrotum for tenderness, swelling, and nodules.
  - Note presence and complete descent of each testicle.
  - Check each testicle for tenderness, swelling, and nodules. Is each freely mobile?
  - Spermatic cord is free of tenderness, swelling, and nodules.
  - No bulging from the inguinal canal or inguinal lymphadenopathy.

Important nursing implications	Abnormal findings
Common clinical findings	Patient teaching

TESTICULAR SELF-EXAMINATION (TSE)

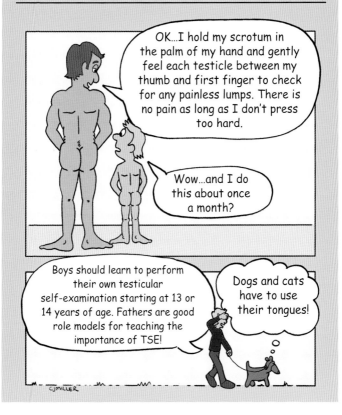

OK...I hold my scrotum in the palm of my hand and gently feel each testicle between my thumb and first finger to check for any painless lumps. There is no pain as long as I don't press too hard.

Wow...and I do this about once a month?

Boys should learn to perform their own testicular self-examination starting at 13 or 14 years of age. Fathers are good role models for teaching the importance of TSE!

Dogs and cats have to use their tongues!

CJMILLER

Assessment at a Glance
Testicular Self-Examination (TSE)

Although the incidence of testicular cancer is relatively low, the TSE is the best way to detect its presence. Testicular cancer occurs in men mostly from ages 15 to 40 years. As with the male genitalia physical assessment, a matter-of-fact approach is best. Much of the TSE can be taught during the physical assessment of the male genitalia. However, the examiner will want to ask for a return demonstration to ensure proficiency.

Boys should be taught this procedure around 13 or 14 years of age. If the father can be the role model, the practice may be more effective and important to the boy. TSE should be performed monthly. (The client may wish to associate it with a monthly bill.)

PROCEDURE

- Warm room and warm hands are best. (Coolness causes the scrotum to contract and shrink.)
- It is best if performed in a warm bath or shower.
- Hold the scrotum in the palm of the hand and look for any abnormalities, masses, nodules, or swelling.
- Roll each testicle between the thumb and first two fingers.
  - Note any tenderness, nodules, masses, swelling, or lesions.
- Gently squeeze the spermatic cord and back edge of each testicle.
- Testicles should be smooth and rubbery.
- Teach client to report any masses, nodules, swelling, pain, or heavy sensations in the scrotum.

ACRONYM

TSE—Helpful to remember when and how to perform a self-examination.
- Timing
- Shower
- Examine

Important nursing implications	Abnormal findings
Common clinical findings	Patient teaching

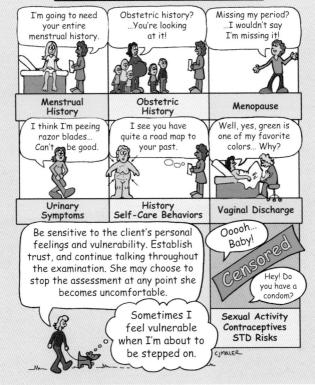

ASSESSMENT OF FEMALE GENITALIA—QUESTIONS

Assessment at a Glance
Assessment of Female Genitalia—Questions

HISTORY

- Menstrual history (menarche to menopause)
- Gravida para—spontaneous or elective abortions
- Sexual satisfaction, activity, and practices (number of partners per year, contraception)
- Oral or anal sex practices; sexually transmitted diseases
- Family history—cancer
- Papanicolaou (PAP) smear—how often and last results
- Genitourinary, renal, reproductive disease or surgery
- Structure and lesions
  - Relating to the vagina; Erythema? Swelling or bulging?
  - Changes associated with straining or lifting?
  - Masses or nodules? Lesions, blisters, ulcers, chancre? Exudate or discharge?
- Urinary pattern and characteristics
  - Careful questioning—symptoms can be hard to describe.
  - Frequent voidings of small amounts? Incontinence? Urgency to void and after voiding?
  - Dribbling before or after voiding or with sneezing or coughing?
  - Urine color, odor, consistency, clarity (dark, foul, cloudy, blood-tinged)?
  - Discharge, pus, oozing (vaginal or urethral)?
- Pain
  - Location, onset, duration, quality, radiation
  - Associated with voiding (before, during, after)?
  - Associated with intercourse (before, during, after)?
  - Associated with menstruation or premenstrual syndrome (PMS)?
  - Other precipitating factors? Itching or burning?
  - Does pain change with movement, lifting, or straining?
  - Radiation of pain to stomach or back?

Important nursing implications	Abnormal findings
Common clinical findings	Patient teaching

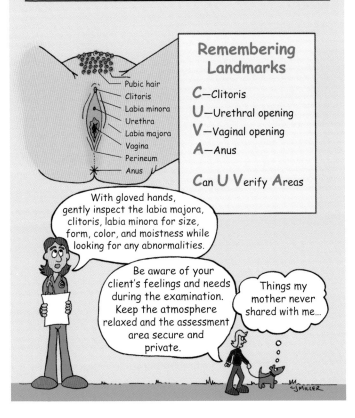

Assessment at a Glance
Assessment of Female Genitalia

The preferable position for the examination is lithotomy. The nurse will want to warn the client before touching her to avoid startling her. Male examiners may wish to have an assistant present for observation.

NORMAL RANGE OF FINDINGS

- Preparation and position; empty bladder
- Inspection
  - Identify CUVA (**c**litoris, **u**rethral opening [slitlike and midline], **v**aginal opening [asymmetrical narrow or large opening], **a**nus).
  - Symmetrical anatomy; hair distribution
  - Discharge? Erythema, lesions, chancres, genital warts?
  - Trauma, episiotomy scar? Hemorrhoids? Vaginal or bladder prolapse?
- Palpation
  - Insert one finger partially into vagina; gently milk urethra.
  - Palpate along each labia majora (Skene's and Bartholin's glands).
    - Labia should be smooth, soft, and homogenous.
    - Separate labia with two fingers; ask the woman to bear down; no bulging is observed in the vaginal walls. Incontinence? Pain?
  - Perineum is firm and muscular.

ABNORMAL FINDINGS

- Inspection
  - Labia asymmetrical; enlarged clitoris, inflammation, erythema, excoriation
  - Altered pigmentation of the skin, hair (infestations)
  - Discharge—foul odor; yellow, white, or bloody
  - Erythema, lesions, chancres, nodules, genital warts
  - Trauma, episiotomy scar; hemorrhoids, vaginal or bladder prolapse
- Palpation
  - Vaginal bulging—cystocele, rectocele, vaginal prolapse
  - Swelling, urethral discharge; pain on palpation, thin perineum

Important nursing implications	Abnormal findings
Common clinical findings	Patient teaching

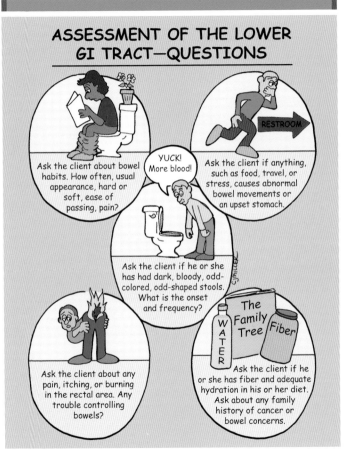

Assessment at a Glance
Assessment of the Lower GI Tract—Questions

HISTORY

- Normal bowel patterns (frequency, consistency, color)
  - Incontinence; explosive bowel movements
- Normal flatus patterns (associated with eating or certain foods)
- Dietary effects on bowel movements
  - Lactose intolerance; food allergies; GI colic reflex
- Medications
  - Enemas, suppositories, laxatives, antidiarrheal medications
  - Narcotics, cholesterol-lowering medications, diabetes medications
- Hydration—number of glasses of water per day
- Bowel diversion (colostomy, colectomy)
- Fissures, fistulas, hemorrhoids
- Anal sex
- Health maintenance screenings—fecal occult blood test, colonoscopy and endoscopy history
- Family history of bowel cancer or concerns
- Other household members with similar symptoms
- Association with pregnancy or menstruation
- Recent travel
- Social concerns (Children may not like defecating anywhere but at home.)
- Appearance and characteristics of stool
  - Any blood or mucus (lower GI issues); black tarry stools (upper GI bleed)
  - Gray stools (hepatic or biliary pathologic condition)
  - Hard, soft, liquid, shreds
- Pain
  - Location, onset, duration, quality, radiation
    - Associated with before, during, or after bowel movement
    - Burning during or after defecation
    - Itching; cramping during or after meals

| Important nursing implications | Abnormal findings |
| Common clinical findings | Patient teaching |

ASSESSMENT OF THE LOWER GI TRACT—RECTAL EXAMINATION

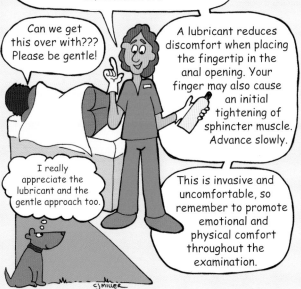

The anus should look moist and hairless, with rough wrinkles and dark pigmentation, and no inflammation.

Can we get this over with??? Please be gentle!

A lubricant reduces discomfort when placing the fingertip in the anal opening. Your finger may also cause an initial tightening of sphincter muscle. Advance slowly.

I really appreciate the lubricant and the gentle approach too.

This is invasive and uncomfortable, so remember to promote emotional and physical comfort throughout the examination.

Assessment at a Glance
Assessment of the Lower GI Tract—Rectal Examination

Provide privacy and warmth as much as possible during this examination. The examiner may want an observer of the opposite sex to witness the examination.

NORMAL RANGE OF FINDINGS

- Preparation and position
  - Prostate examination—Male client bends over the end of a table with legs apart to shoulder width.
  - Female—Assumes lithotomy position. Male—Assumes left lying position.
- Inspection
  - Anus is closed, moist, and hairless with rough wrinkles.
  - Wrinkles and ridges are symmetrical in size.
  - Is usually darker in pigmentation; no inflammation is observed.
  - Ask client to hold breath and bear down; no protrusion or fissures are present.
- Palpation
  - Don gloves; place drop (marble size) of water-soluble jelly on the finger.
  - Touch the pad of the finger to the anus (should tighten then relax).
  - Slowly advance finger into anus (no pain).
  - Rotate finger, feeling sphincter all the way around (smooth, no pain).
  - Client squeezes finger without pain.
  - Advance finger further in the rectum, palpating the walls. It should be nontender.
  - No openings, breaks, or bumps have developed in the rectal wall.
  - Rectal wall is smooth and nontender.
  - Stool is brown, no blood or black tarry stool are present.

ABNORMAL FINDINGS

- Inspection
  - Tuft of hair, dimpling near the coccyx; inflammation, erythema
  - Fissures, hemorrhoids

Important nursing implications	Abnormal findings
Common clinical findings	Patient teaching

ASSESSMENT OF THE NEUROLOGIC SYSTEM—QUESTIONS

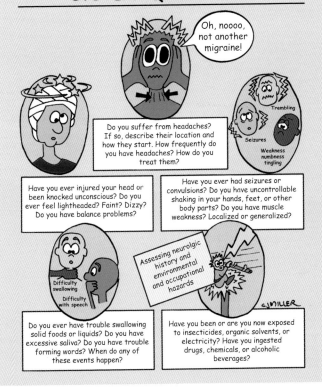

Assessment at a Glance
Assessment of the Neurologic System—Questions

HISTORY

- Medications used for the treatment of:
  - Parkinson's disease, Alzheimer's disease, seizures
  - Stroke, myasthenia gravis, multiple sclerosis, other neurologic agents
- Head injury or other central nervous system trauma
- Changes in ability to concentrate, hallucinations, delusions, forgetfulness
- Menstrual history, menopause, pregnancy history
- Changes in bowel and bladder functions
- Medical history (stroke, epilepsy, emotional disorders)
- Significant life changes (trauma, loss, abuse)
- Bedwetting, family history of seizures, cerebral palsy, muscular dystrophy
- Occupational hazard (military service, chemicals)
- Drug abuse (alcoholism, hallucinogens); recent travel, camping
- Co-morbidity (hepatitis, renal failure)

SYMPTOMS REPORTED

- Mentation
  - Change in personality (anger, more emotional, flat affect)
  - Change in alertness (alert, lethargic, obtunded, stupor, comatose)
- Communication
  - Receptive or expressive aphasia; dysphasia (difficulty speaking)
- Motor
  - Tremors at rest and intentional, twitch, tick
  - Stiffness, rigidity, difficulty in both initiating and stopping movement
  - Coordination, dysphagia (difficulty swallowing)
- Sensation
  - Paresthesias, burning or tingling, nausea
  - Numbness, no sensation, balance problems
- Pain
  - Location, onset, duration, quality, radiation
  - Patterns in pain presentation, causes, and relief

ASSESSMENT OF THE NEUROLOGIC SYSTEM—TOOLS OF THE TRADE

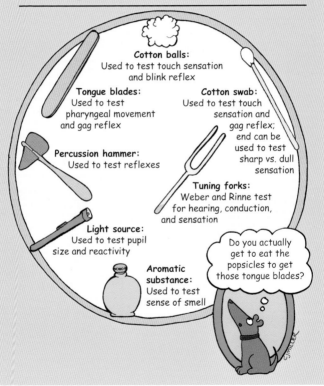

Assessment of the Neurologic System—Tools of the Trade

- Ask the client whether he or she has any questions before using the tools. Younger children may prefer to handle the tools, which will be useful in helping alleviate anxiety in the child and facilitating cooperation. Explain to the client the purpose of the tools.
- Cotton balls—Used to test light touch and the corneal blink reflex. Throw the cotton away after use. Do not use cotton on the cornea after it has been used for light touch.
- Cotton swab (cotton-tip applicator)—Used to test light touch. Can be used for testing sharp or dull sensation (some may prefer to break the swab in half for testing sharp and dull sensations). The clean swab can also be used for testing the gag reflex. Ensure that the jagged edge is used gently to prevent breaking the skin.
- Tuning fork (128 or 256 Hz)—Used for the Rinne and Weber tests to assess hearing; can also be used to test vibratory sensation.
- Aromatic substance—Used to test smell (olfactory nerve). Coffee and vanilla extract may be used.
- Light source—Can be a penlight, flashlight, otoscope, or ophthalmoscope. It is used for testing the papillary light reflex and the oculomotor system (corneal light reflex).
- Percussion hammer—Used to test deep tendon reflexes.
- Tongue blade—Used to test gag reflex and palate and uvula movement. If the tongue blade is broken in half, then it may be used to test sharp and dull sensations. Ensure that the jagged edge is used gently to prevent breaking the skin.
- Although these tools do not need to be sterile, they do need to be clean.
- Suggested sequence for conducting the complete neurologic examination:
  1. Mental status
  2. Cranial nerves
  3. Motor system
  4. Sensory system
  5. Reflexes

Important nursing implications	Abnormal findings
Common clinical findings	Patient teaching

ASSESSMENT OF THE NEUROLOGIC SYSTEM—CRANIAL NERVES 1-6

Olfactory Nerve I

Check each nostril for occlusion. With the client's eyes closed, place a distinct aroma near each nonoccluded nostril.

Optic Nerve II

Check ocular fundus and optic disc for color, shape, and size.

Oculomotor, Trochlear, and Abducens Nerves III, IV, VI

Check pupils with a light for reaction and accommodation. Assess extraocular movements and eye oscillation.

Trigeminal Nerve V

Ask the client to clench his or her teeth. Palpate the temporal and masseter muscles.

My friend, Murphy... He has nerves. He's not afraid of anything!

Ophthalmic

Maxillary

Mandibular

Use a piece of cotton to touch areas of the face lightly. Ask the client to tell you when he or she feels the cotton.

CJMILLER

```
━━━━━━━━━━━━ Assessment at a Glance ━━━━━━━━━━━━
```

Assessment of the Neurologic System—Cranial Nerves 1-6

- Preparation and position
  - Ask the client to sit on the examination table for this part of the neurologic examination. Provide warmth; limit distractions.
  - Use only clean equipment. (Don't reuse cotton swabs.)
- Olfactory nerve (I)
  - Check for bilateral patency.
  - With eyes closed, test each nostril with a distinct aroma (coffee, peppermint, vanilla). Try to use a different aroma on each side.
- Optic nerve (II)
  - Using the ophthalmoscope, check the optic disc for color, shape, and size.
  - Check visual acuity (Snellen eye chart).
  - Check peripheral vision (visual fields by confrontation).
- Oculomotor, trochlear, abducens nerves (III, IV, VI)
  - Pupillary light reflex
    - Darken room (opens and dilates pupils).
    - Client looks at a distant object (opens and dilates pupils).
    - Light source should see direct reflex (same side pupil constricts) and consensual light reflex (simultaneous constriction of other pupil).
    - PERRLA—**P**upils are **E**qual and **R**ound; they **R**eact to **L**ight; **A**ccommodation occurs.
- Accommodation
  - Client looks far (pupil dilates); looks near (3 inches) (pupil constricts).
    - Extraocular movements are examined.
    - Client follows the nurse's finger or pen to the six cardinal fields of gaze.
    - Nystagmus is only seen with the eyes looking at extreme lateral gaze.
- Trigeminal nerve (V)
  - Motor—Palpate the temporal and masseter muscles; clench teeth.
    - Muscles contract strongly and symmetrically.
  - Sensory—Using cotton, bilaterally assess touch in three areas of the face (forehead, maxilla, chin).

Important nursing implications	Abnormal findings
Common clinical findings	Patient teaching

ASSESSMENT OF THE NEUROLOGIC SYSTEM—CRANIAL NERVES 7-12

Facial Nerve VII
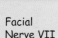
Assess mobility and symmetry of the client's facial features. Ask the client to frown, smile, show teeth, and puff cheeks.

Acoustic (Vestibulocochlear) Nerve VIII

Can you hear me now?
Use the whispered voice test and a tuning fork to assess the client's hearing and acuity.

Glossopharyngeal and Vagus Nerves IX, X

Gag
Check the gag reflex. Watch for movement of the uvula, soft palate, and tonsils.

Spinal Accessory Nerve XI

Check the sternomastoid and trapezius muscles for equal strength by asking the client to turn his or her head against resistance.

I get nervous when it comes to cats...

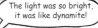
The light was so bright, it was like dynamite!

Assess the tongue for wasting or tremors. Listen to words for clarity, tone, and distinctness. Ask the client to stick out his or her tongue.

Hypoglossal Nerve XII

CJMILLER

Assessment at a Glance

Assessment of the Neurologic System—Cranial Nerves 7-12

- Preparation and position
  - Ask the client to sit on the examination table for this part of the neurologic examination.
  - Provide warmth, and limit distractions.
  - Use only clean equipment (do not reuse cotton swabs).
- Facial nerve (VII)
  - Smile, frown, squeeze eyes shut, and keep closed against resistance; puff out cheeks (symmetry).
- Acoustic or vestibulocochlear nerve (VIII)
  - Client's speech is clear.
  - At 1 to 2 feet, whisper phrase and ask client to repeat.
  - Ask client to occlude opposite ear.
  - Conduct Weber and Rinne tests—Sound is heard equally in both ears.
- Glossopharyngeal and vagus nerves (IX, X)
  - Gag—Visualize uvula and soft palate rising symmetrically on both sides; tonsillar pillars move medially.
- Spinal accessory nerve (XI)
  - Assess sternomastoid and trapezius muscle strength.
    - Against resistance—Shrug shoulders, turn head left and right and move ear to shoulder left to right.
- Hypoglossal nerve (XII)
  - Stick out tongue, point left, point right, push out left cheek, and push out right cheek.
  - No wasting or atrophy is observed; tongue is midline when sticking straight out.

| Important nursing implications | Abnormal findings |
| Common clinical findings | Patient teaching |

ASSESSMENT OF THE NEUROLOGIC SYSTEM—INSPECTION AND MOVEMENT

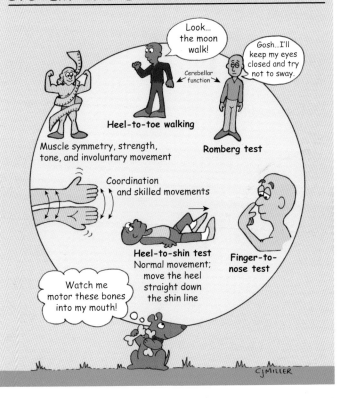

Assessment of the Neurologic System—Inspection and Movement

- Cerebellar function
  - Tandem walking—Client walks heel to toe without losing balance.
  - Romberg test—Feet are together, eyes are closed with arms at side for 20 seconds (no falling or spreading feet to catch balance, may normally observe a small amount of swaying). Positive Romberg test—Client falls.
- Coordination
  - Finger to nose—Arms are held out to the sides, eyes are closed. Client is able to touch nose with finger from both hands.
  - Move heel down to shin—While sitting or lying down without looking, client is able to run the heel of one foot down the front of the opposite shin.
  - Rapid alternating movements
    - Finger thumb—While looking, client touches the thumb to each of the four fingers quickly; can repeat with the other hand.
    - Hand flip flop—While looking and with both hands on lap, client flip flops or turns hands over on thighs and is able to keep repeating quickly.
- Musculature
  - Tone to muscles is not being used (symmetrical).
  - Hand grasp; push and pull against resistance.
  - Feet—Push toes down, pull toes to ceiling against resistance.
  - No twitching, ticks, or tremors are observed.

Important nursing implications	Abnormal findings
Common clinical findings	Patient teaching

ASSESSMENT OF THE NEUROLOGIC SYSTEM—TESTING SENSES AND REFLEXES

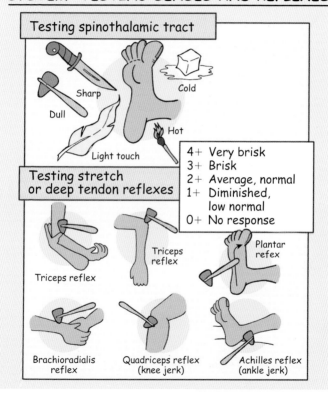

Testing spinothalamic tract

Sharp

Dull

Cold

Hot

Light touch

4+ Very brisk
3+ Brisk
2+ Average, normal
1+ Diminished,
     low normal
0+ No response

Testing stretch
or deep tendon reflexes

Triceps reflex

Triceps reflex

Plantar refex

Brachioradialis reflex

Quadriceps reflex (knee jerk)

Achilles reflex (ankle jerk)

Assessment at a Glance

Assessment of the Neurologic System—Testing Senses and Reflexes

The ability to sense sharp, dull, light touch, and hot and cold is very important. This ability offers the client protective capability as they move around in the environment. The deep tendon reflex (stretch reflex) is an indication of the health of the central nervous system and intact reflex arc.

- Spinothalamic function
  - Eyes should be closed for sensory testing.
  - Vibration—Use a 128 or 256 Hz tuning fork.
    - Instruct the client to say when he or she feels the vibration and when the vibration is no longer felt.
    - Tap the tines of the tuning fork on the edge of a table or on the ball of the hand.
    - Place the tuning fork stem on the distal joint of a finger or toe. Wait for indication that the client feels the vibration.
    - Stop the vibration by gently grasping both tines.
    - Client is able to indicate when vibration is felt and when it is no longer present.
  - Assess sharp and dull sensations with a broken tongue blade or a cotton-tip applicator.
  - Assess hot and cold sensations with two test tubes (one with warm water, another with cold water).
  - Assess light touch with a cotton wisp.
- Deep tendon reflex (stretch reflex)
  - Use percussion hammer at wrist.
  - Palpate the muscle being assessed if possible.
  - Ratings: +1 or +2 (both 0 and +3 may very rarely be a normal variation; +4 abnormal); symmetry is observed.
  - May need a distraction.
  - Hangs extremity similar to "spaghetti."
  - Babinski test—Plantar flexion (except in the infant) is assessed.
  - Positive Babinski test—dorsiflexion and toe fanning (except in the infant)

Important nursing implications	Abnormal findings
Common clinical findings	Patient teaching

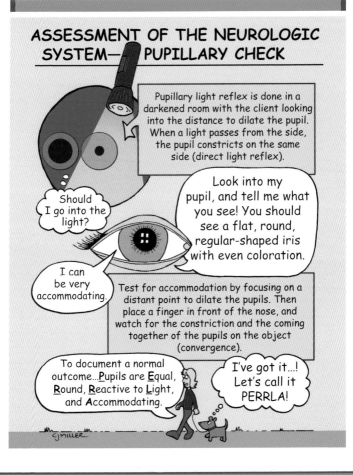

Assessment at a Glance

Assessment of the Neurologic System—Pupillary Check

- Pupillary light reflex
  - Note pupil size, symmetry, shape; iris color, iris symmetry, and iris shape.
  - Darken the room to open and dilate the pupils.
  - Client looks at a distant object to open and dilate the pupil.
  - Light source should be focused; only one eye is "shined" at a time.
  - Direct light reflex response is a constriction (miosis) in the eye being shined.
  - Consensual light reflex response is when the opposite pupil constricts, when shining a light in the other eye.
- Accommodation
  - Client looks far; "Please look at the wall over there" (dilation).
  - Client then looks near (3 inches); "Please look at my finger" (constriction).
- PERRLA—**P**upils **E**qual, **R**ound, **R**eact to **L**ight, and **A**ccommodation

ABNORMAL FINDINGS

- Pupillary light reflex
  - Pupils are pinpoint, constricted, and fixed (miosis).
    - Could be drug related, central nervous system related, or an indication of inflammation of the iris.
  - Pupils are overly dilated and fixed (mydriasis).
    - Could be drug related; may indicate central nervous system injury, acute glaucoma, or sympathetic stimulation.
  - Anisocoria—Unequal pupils are observed.
    - May be a normal variation or an indication of central nervous system disease.
  - Pupils do not respond to light; pupils demonstrate a sluggish response.
  - Pupils respond asymmetrically (no consensual light reflex).
- Accommodation
  - Asymmetrical pupil sizes can be an indication of closed head injury.
  - Constricted pupils can be a sign of drug overdose or toxicity.

Important nursing implications	Abnormal findings
Common clinical findings	Patient teaching

ASSESSMENT OF PREGNANCY—THREE Ps

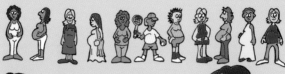

RESUMPTIVE SIGNS
- Amenorrhea
- Nausea
- Fatigue
- Breast tenderness
- Urinary frequency
- Quickening

ROBABLE SIGNS
- Enlarged uterus
- Positive pregnancy test
- Chadwick's sign
- Hegar's sign
- Goodell's sign

OSITIVE SIGNS
- Fetal heart rate
- Visualization by ultrasound

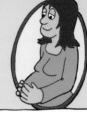

Clients have different beliefs, lifestyles, and backgrounds. Each pregnancy is just as unique. The nurse's approach should make care, kindness, and consideration the hallmark words in assessment.

Dogs like care and kindness too!

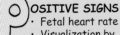

Assessment at a Glance
Assessment of Pregnancy—Three Ps

Three Ps can help the nurse remember the signs and symptoms of pregnancy: **presumptive**, **probable**, and **positive**. The prenatal visit is a good time to teach the client the signs and symptoms of pregnancy.

- Presumptive (signs reported by the client—subjective findings)
  - Amenorrhea
  - Nausea
  - Urinary frequency
  - Uterus compressing the bladder
  - Fatigue
  - Breast tenderness, fullness, increased pigmentation of areola, precolostrum discharge
  - Quickening
    - Mother feels the movement of the baby (could be confused with gas or abdominal peristalsis).
- Probable (detected by examination—objective findings)
  - Enlarged uterus
  - Ballottement (fetal- or uterine-floating type of movement)
  - Positive pregnancy blood or urine tests
  - Midabdominal distension
  - Hegar's sign—softening of the lower uterine segment
  - Chadwick's sign—bluish discoloration of the vagina
  - Goodell's sign—softening of the cervical lip
- Positive (clear proof)
  - Fetal heart rate (use of a Doppler ultrasound stethoscope)
    - Some fetal heart monitors are a simple speaker and the nurse manually counts; others are more complex and the monitor will display the count.
  - Visualization by ultrasound
  - Fetal movements felt by examiner

| Important nursing implications | Abnormal findings |
| Common clinical findings | Patient teaching |

ASSESSMENT OF PREGNANCY—INSPECTION

Use all your senses during the assessment to collect accurate verbal and nonverbal information.

Overall Approach and Inspection

Look for chloasma, cesarean surgical line, striae gravidarum (stretch marks), linea nigra, and spider veins.

Skin Inspection

Check thyroid area for swelling. Check mucous membranes for color, moisture, and smoothness.

Mouth and Neck

Observe the breast for:
- Colostrum
- Distended veins
- Striae gravidarum
- Enlarged, darkened, erect nipples
- Secondary areolar changes

Breast Changes

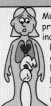

Murmurs may be present as a result of increased blood volume. Lungs should remain clear. Shortness of breath may be present in the third trimester because of upward pressure.

Heart and Lung Sounds

I have six nipples... but I don't think they work.

CJMILLER

Assessment at a Glance
Assessment of Pregnancy—Inspection

SKIN

- Chloasma—mask of pregnancy; Cesarean delivery scar
- Striae gravidarum—stretch marks
- Linea nigra—hyperpigmented line centralized over abdomen from sternal notch to symphysis pubis
- Spider veins—vascular veins on upper body
- Edema (especially in lower extremities)

MOUTH AND NECK

- Color and moisture—mucosa, lips, skin (cyanosis)
- Thyroid—symmetrical, nonpalpable

BREASTS

- Colostrum may be expressed throughout pregnancy.
- Nipples are enlarged, darkened, and erect.
- Secondary areolar changes develop. Areolae are usually larger and darker with mottling around each.
- Remind the client to continue monthly BSE during pregnancy.
  - The hormones of pregnancy might encourage the growth of cancer; therefore the woman should continue monitoring.

HEART AND LUNG SOUNDS

- Assess for murmurs.
  - Increased blood volume may lead to a soft systolic murmur.
  - Women with heart disease before pregnancy should be closely monitored.
- Lung sounds should remain clear.
  - Dyspnea may occur, especially in the third trimester.

PERIPHERAL VASCULATURE

- Varicose veins—Discuss lower extremity exercises to decrease chances of clot formation.
- Hemorrhoids—Caused by pressure on the pelvic veins.

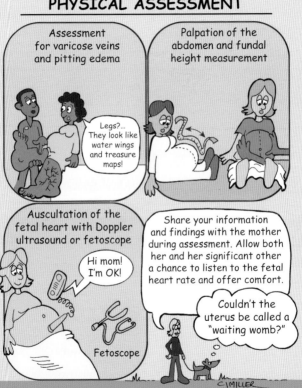

ASSESSMENT OF PREGNANCY— PHYSICAL ASSESSMENT

Assessment for varicose veins and pitting edema

Legs?... They look like water wings and treasure maps!

Palpation of the abdomen and fundal height measurement

Auscultation of the fetal heart with Doppler ultrasound or fetoscope

Hi mom! I'm OK!

Fetoscope

Share your information and findings with the mother during assessment. Allow both her and her significant other a chance to listen to the fetal heart rate and offer comfort.

Couldn't the uterus be called a "waiting womb?"

Assessment at a Glance
Assessment of Pregnancy—Physical Assessment

The nurse should explain the procedures and their purposes as the examination progresses.

- Periphery
  - Varicose veins
  - Edema
    - Tends to be worse in the third trimester.
    - Tends to be worse later in the day.
- Abdominal
  - Palpation—Uterus is usually nontender; abdominal muscles become softer with each pregnancy.
    - Identify the fundus by placing both hands on either side of the uterus and walking hands toward the woman's rib cage.
    - Braxton-Hicks contractions can be palpated, whereas the uterus usually contracts and rises (mild = tip of the nose; moderate = chin; hard = forehead; can be used as a guide to determine strength of contraction).
  - Fundal height measurement—Measure from the superior border of the symphysis pubis to the fundus.
  - After 20 weeks, the fundal height in centimeters should equal the weeks in the pregnancy.
  - Leopold's maneuvers—Performed during the third trimester to determine fetal lie, position, presentation, and status of engagement.
- Fetal
  - Auscultation—Slower sounds may be the placental or maternal pulse (maternal souffle—soft swishing sound of placenta receiving pulse of maternal arterial blood).
    - Doppler ultrasound—Normal fetal rate is 120 to 160 beats per minute.
    - Fetoscope

| Important nursing implications | Abnormal findings |
| Common clinical findings | Patient teaching |

ASSESSMENT OF INFANTS (BIRTH TO 1 YEAR)

Cognitive Development

Physical Development

Erikson's Trust vs. Mistrust

Birth to 1 Year

Motor Development

I love the smell of baby's breath.

Cerebral Cortex Growth

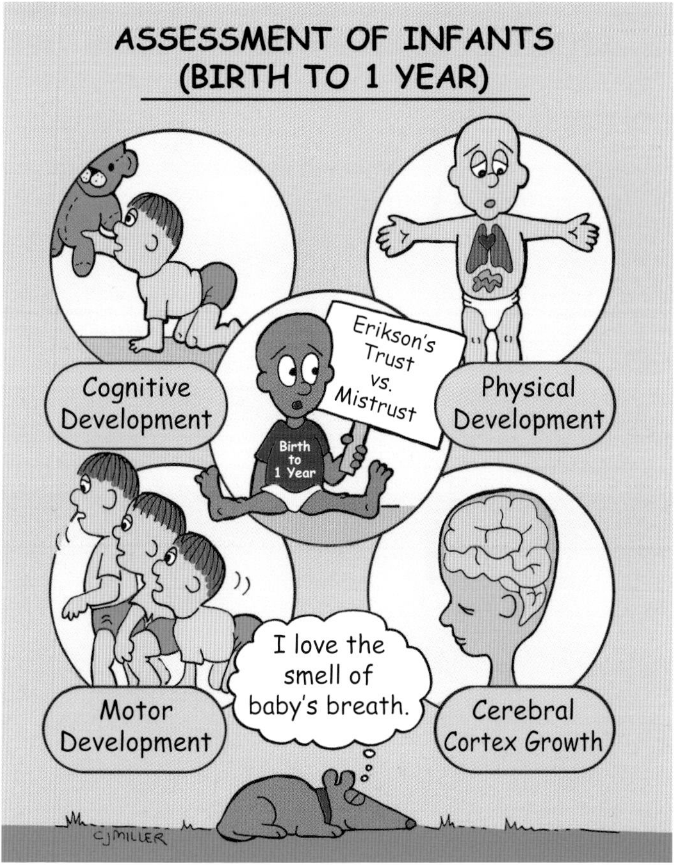

============ Assessment at a Glance ============
Assessment of Infants (Birth to 1 Year)

Although some variability may exist, an infant will double his or her weight in 6 months and triple the birth weight by 12 months.

- Cognitive development
  - 1 month—Reflexes are the primary drive.
  - 2 months—Visual tracking is noted.
  - 4 months—Hands are put together, audible tracking is observed.
  - 6 months—Can adjust posture, scans for parent, recognizes name.
  - 10 months—Explores for toys, enjoys books.
- Organ systems
  - Attempt auscultation without disturbing the child (while sleeping, feeding). May ask the parent to continue holding the child during this part of the examination.
  - Systolic murmurs are common in children and are not considered a pathologic condition if the murmurs do not radiate and can change with position change.
  - Stranger anxiety after 6 months can make assessment difficult.
  - Turgor is important for identifying dehydration (examination can be performed on abdomen).
  - Lymph nodes that are firm, tender, warm, and in the left supraclavicular notch are important variations to note and explore further.
  - Anterior fontanel closes between 12 and 18 months; posterior fontanel closes at 2 months.
- Visual acuity
  - 1 month—20/100; 2 months—visual tracking is noted; 4 months—20/80; 6 months—focus on small objects; 10 months—20/40
- Cerebral cortex growth
  - Information from parent can provide important clues about cerebral cortex development and the infant's response to stimuli (auditory, visual, tactile).
- Motor development
  - Birth to 4 months—May roll over, voluntary grasp reflex.
  - 4 to 7 months—Rolls over, sits alone at 6 months, crawls.
  - 8 to 12 months—Stands alone, cruises around furniture.

ASSESSMENT OF TODDLERS (1 TO 3 YEARS)

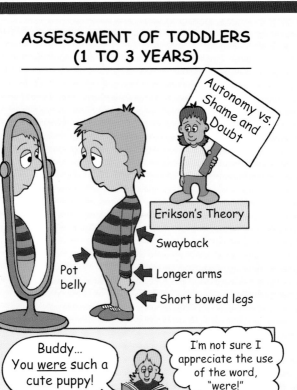

Assessment at a Glance
Assessment of Toddlers (1 to 3 Years)

- Cognitive development
  - Toddler is curious about most aspects of the world (tactile, auditory, visual).
  - This curiosity allows the toddler to absorb large amounts of information that facilitate growth.
  - Parent will provide valuable information about the toddler's actions and interactions that can provide valuable health assessment data.
  - The Denver Developmental Screening Test II (DDST-II) is an important tool for the nurse to identify developmental milestones up to 6 years of age.
    - The DDST-II includes assessment of interpersonal interactions, fine and gross motor skills, and language development.
- Organ systems
  - Distracting the toddler with other tools or toys may facilitate the physical assessment.
  - A calm, slow approach may facilitate cooperation.
  - Musculoskeletal system should progress constantly:
    - 12 months—walking
    - 18-24 months—climbing stairs, running
    - 36 months—jumping, beginning purposeful drawing
  - Toddler's physique—protuberant abdomen, swayback, long arms, short bowed legs
- Visual acuity
  - 18 months—20/40
  - 36 months—20/20
- Erikson's theory
  - Autonomy vs. shame and doubt
  - Autonomy includes control of the environment, interactions, and body functions.
  - Although avoiding feelings of shame and doubt is part of this stage, the toddler may learn to adapt to some of these feelings.
  - Large emphasis is placed on potty training in this stage.

| Important nursing implications | Abnormal findings |
| Common clinical findings | Patient teaching |

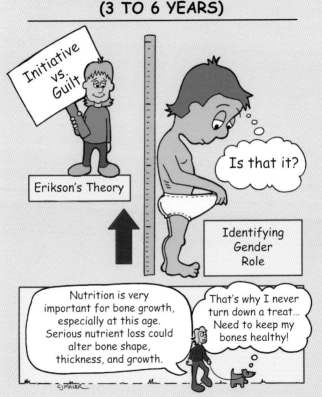

Assessment at a Glance
Assessment of Preschoolers (3 to 6 Years)

- Cognitive development
  - Begins to use adjectives as speech improves to intelligible words.
  - Begins dressing self.
  - Likes to assist with activities of daily living (ADLs).
- Organ systems
  - Allowing the child to handle some of the tools safely may facilitate the physical assessment.
  - A calm, slow approach may facilitate cooperation.
  - Growth should be closely monitored on a growth curve and chart. Different charts exist for boys and girls.
    - Obesity should be addressed if the child is over the eighty-fifth percentile for the body mass index (BMI).
  - Auditory acuity should be assessed with reports of inattentiveness or distractibility.
  - Musculoskeletal system should progress constantly:
    - 36 months—jumping, beginning purposeful drawing
    - 4 to 5 years—hopping on one foot, drawing, writing, throwing, kicking
- Visual acuity
  - 36 months—20/20
  - Tumbling E (Snellen E) type chart—The legs on the letter E point in different directions.
  - HOTV chart—The child holds a board with H-O-T-V on it and points to the letter seen at a distance.
  - Picture chart—Common pictures are used.
  - Visual acuity should be assessed with reports of inattentiveness, distractibility, and headaches.
- Erikson's theory
  - Initiative vs. guilt
  - Gender role identity and goal-oriented initiative begins.
  - Play becomes both imaginative and competitive.

Important nursing implications	Abnormal findings
Common clinical findings	Patient teaching

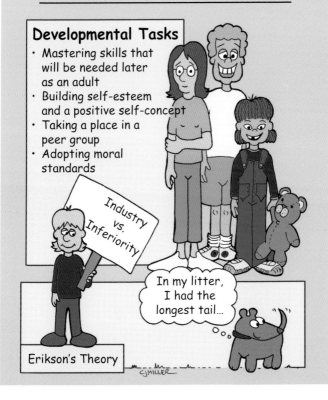

ASSESSMENT OF SCHOOL-AGE CHILDREN (6 TO 12 YEARS)

Developmental Tasks
- Mastering skills that will be needed later as an adult
- Building self-esteem and a positive self-concept
- Taking a place in a peer group
- Adopting moral standards

Industry vs. Inferiority

In my litter, I had the longest tail...

Erikson's Theory

Assessment at a Glance
Assessment of School-Age Children (6 to 12 Years)

- Cognitive development
  - Can use thinking to experience the world.
  - Begins to understand calculation with numbers and sequencing.
  - Begins to think outside of him or herself and realizes that many concepts are multifactorial.
  - The occurrence of puberty and development really distorts age-related levels into preadolescence. Children become individualized in their growth and development.
- Organ systems
  - Allowing the child to handle some of the tools safely may facilitate physical assessment.
  - Address the child, as well as the parent.
  - Encourage the child's participation in the assessment.
  - Growth should be closely monitored on a growth curve and chart. Different charts exist for boys and girls.
    - Obesity should be addressed if the child is over the eighty-fifth percentile for the body mass index (BMI).
  - Auditory and visual acuity should be assessed with reports of inattentiveness, distractibility, emotional changes, or headaches.
  - Musculoskeletal system should progress constantly, although growth rates may affect coordination and strength fluctuation.
  - Reassure the child as he or she becomes aware of the nurse's reactions and nonverbal messages.
- Erikson's theory
  - Industry vs. inferiority
    - Realizes that not everyone can be *good* at everything.
  - As the child develops emotionally, he or she may adopt a first best friend and potentially develop an interest in someone of the opposite sex.
  - Building self-esteem and a positive self-concept are important.
  - Becomes a part of peer groups.

| Important nursing implications | Abnormal findings |
| Common clinical findings | Patient teaching |

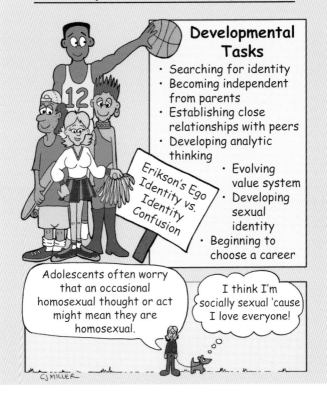

ASSESSMENT OF ADOLESCENTS (12 TO 19 YEARS)

Assessment of Adolescents (12 to 19 Years)

- Cognitive development
  - Abstract thinking becomes common as the person's understanding is not limited to concrete reality.
  - Scientific reasoning may become more prominent in academic and non-academic exercises.
  - Analytical thinking starts to help the development of personal values.
  - Is able to deal more with hypothetical situations.
- Organ systems
  - The adolescent needs clear information during the physical assessment part of the examination. He or she needs to be treated with respect and given accurate information. Nurses should clearly understand the legal boundaries set by their organizations and states related to information release to parents.
  - Growth spurts occur in girls at approximately 12 years of age and in boys at approximately 14 years of age (great variations can occur).
  - Conflict can arise as the adolescent attempts to create personal identity in a body that is constantly and rapidly changing.
  - Development of sex characteristics earlier or later than peers can cause stress. Good health is generally exhibited.
  - Important risks include accidents, sexually transmitted diseases, drug and alcohol abuse, pregnancy, and obesity.
  - Psychologic issues (depression, anorexia, obesity) can affect physiologic health.
- Erikson's theory
  - Ego identity vs. identity confusion
- Morals are developed. Makes a career choice.
- Becomes a part of peer groups.
- Sexual identity—Concern may develop in the adolescent if feelings of homosexuality arise.

| Important nursing implications | Abnormal findings |
| Common clinical findings | Patient teaching |

ASSESSMENT IN EARLY ADULTHOOD (20 TO 40 YEARS)

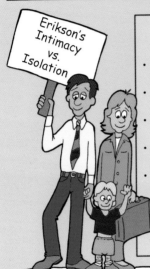

Erikson's Intimacy vs. Isolation

Developmental Tasks

- Growing independent from parents' home and care
- Establishing a career or vocation
- Forming intimate bonds; choosing a mate
- Learning to cooperate in a marriage relationship
- Setting up and managing a household
  - Assuming civic duties
  - Parenting
  - Forming a meaningful philosophy of life

Stress can break down our healthy body. We replace our healthy diets with fast food and sugars. It is important to exercise regularly.

I chase my tail in circles to get my daily exercise.

CJMILLER

Assessment at a Glance

Assessment in Early Adulthood (20 to 40 Years)

After the turbulence of adolescence ends, the young adult becomes better suited to adapt to society. He or she is more able to "see the big picture" and assimilate into mainstream culture. Self-centered tendencies become less prominent.

- Cognitive development
  - Many young adults continue in educational tracks.
  - Some struggle with unemployment and sense of purpose.
  - Some struggle with a lack of access to education.
  - Work is important because of the connection to ego identity.
- Organ systems
  - The young adult is at maximal health and strength.
  - Many health issues come from poor lifestyle choices that include sedentary lifestyle, poor diet, and excess stress (employment, relationships).
  - Reproduction becomes an interest to many.
  - Sexually transmitted diseases remain a major concern.
  - Testicular cancer is at its highest rate in young male adults.
- Erikson's theory
  - Intimacy vs. isolation
  - Self-identity becomes established.
  - Gains independence from parents.
  - Career or vocation is established.
  - Intimate bonds and choosing a mate are important.
  - Operating in a long-term relationship is learned.
  - Home and household are established—Periods of transition and reformulating are common. More exploration happens with those in their 20s, whereas those in their 30s achieve more resolution.
  - Establishes a social group.
  - Assumes civic duties.
  - Becomes a parent.
  - Formulates a philosophy of life.

Important nursing implications	Abnormal findings
Common clinical findings	Patient teaching

ASSESSMENT IN MIDDLE ADULTHOOD (40 TO 60 YEARS)

Help! I think I've lost my menses! Why is it so hot? I'm roasting!

A woman's body goes through many changes during her life from 40 years old on.

Menopause starts around 40 to 50 years of age:
- Changes in cycle duration and quality of flow
- Cessation of flow
  - Changes in cervical mucosa
  - Decreases in estrogen and progesterone
  - Hot flashes
  - Mood swings

First, my prostate cuts off my urine flow, and now I can't stand up... What's next?

The reproductive system in men also begins to degenerate between ages 40 and 50 years but less abruptly. Men have issues with:
- Decreased testosterone
- Decreased sperm and semen production
- Prostate enlargement
- Erectile dysfunction

Middle age is considered the sandwich generation because those in this age group find themselves taking care of their own children while caring for aging parents.

I prefer my sandwiches with roast beef and mustard!

CJMILLER

Assessment at a Glance
Assessment in Middle Adulthood (40 to 60 Years)

The middle adult often becomes the caretaker for multiple generations. This generation is at the peak of vocational responsibility.

- Cognitive development
  - May return to school and seek second degree or career.
  - Life experiences of this group allow for very rich learning interactions, which includes a sense of humor and responsibility all at the same time.
  - The application of learning and knowledge becomes important, and deep social meaning may be sought.
- Organ systems
  - Many changes occur that are related to the reproductive system.
  - Female—menopause-related changes
    - Cessation of menses; irregular cycles and duration
    - Hot flashes (Some refer to these as a "power surges.")
    - Changes in cervical mucosa; decreases in estrogen and progesterone
    - Mood swings
  - Male—sexual identity–related changes that are less abrupt than those occurring with female middle adults
    - Prostate enlargement
    - Erectile dysfunction—decreased testosterone
    - Decreased sperm and semen production; hair loss
  - Certain health screenings become important in this stage:
    - Colon, breast, and prostate cancer
- Erikson's theory
  - Generativity vs. stagnation
  - Accepts physiologic changes.
  - Conducts vocational self-analysis (affirms career or makes a midcourse correction).
  - Hobby and leisure activities become more important.
  - Parents and children are changing with increased age.
  - Affirms spousal relationship or the lack thereof.

Important nursing implications	Abnormal findings
Common clinical findings	Patient teaching

ASSESSMENT IN OLDER ADULTHOOD (60 TO 80 YEARS)

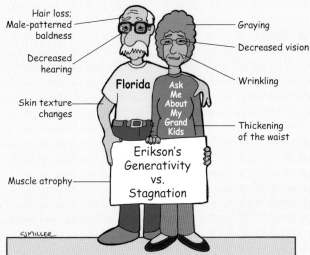

Developmental Tasks

- Accepting and adjusting to physical changes
- Adjusting to retirement and change in income
- Conducting a life review
- Developing hobby and leisure activities
- Helping children search for identity
- Preparing for death of self and spouse

Assessment at a Glance
Assessment in Older Adulthood (60 to 80 Years)

Many older adults are geographically separated from their families and are still very active in their careers. The economic state of many older adults leaves them in dire situations that require the nurse to assess multiple facets of their life simultaneously.

- Cognitive development
  - Many in this age group realize no decline or change in cognitive functioning.
    - Changes in cognitive function are multifactorial and can be the result of:
      - Illness; heredity; mental activity; social interactions; sensory deprivation and functioning
  - Assessment in cognitive functioning—the Mini-Mental Status Examination
- Organ systems
  - Physical assessment in this stage of life often takes longer. Older adult clients have more information to provide, and their cases may be complex. If the nurse tries to rush this assessment, not only will important information be lost, but the therapeutic relationship will also be hampered.
  - Sensory
    - Presbycusis and presbyopia
    - Glaucoma, cataracts, macular degeneration
  - Integument
    - Diet leading to dehydration (poor skin turgor, fragile skin)
    - Wrinkled skin; graying hair
  - Multiple and chronic diseases
    - Polypharmacy; lower income and higher medical costs
- Erikson's theory
  - Ego integrity vs. despair
  - Accepts physiologic changes. Reminisces (positive reflection).
  - Develops a sense of wisdom.
  - Accepts successes and disappointments.
  - Develops a fear of death or accepts that death is nearing.
  - Desires relationships with younger generations.

Important nursing implications	Abnormal findings
Common clinical findings	Patient teaching

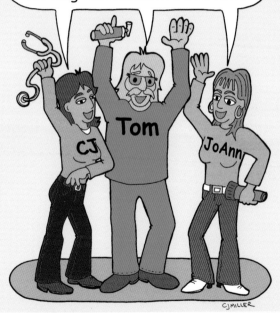